CW00695116

WALL PILATES WORKOUTS FOR WOMEN

TRANSFORM YOUR BODY IN JUST 28 DAYS

STEP-BY-STEP EXERCISES WITH REAL PHOTOS TO TONE GLUTES, SHAPE ABS, STRENGTHEN CORE, AND ACHIEVE PERFECT POSTURE

SERENA WALLIS

TABLE OF CONTENT

Copyright 2023 by Serena Wallis – All right reserved

This publication is protected by copyright. No part of this publication may be distributed or reproduced, including photocopying or other methods, without a signed permission of the owner. However, brief quotations, including critical reviews and other noncommercial uses permitted by copyright law, may be used with proper citation.

The contents of this book are intended solely for general information purposes. Although we do our best to ensure that the information in this book is accurate and current, we cannot guarantee its completeness, reliability, or suitability for any purpose. The information in the book is provided without any warranties. Any decision you make based on this information is at your own risk.

We shall not be held responsible for any loss or damage, including but not limited to indirect or consequential loss or damage, arising from the use of this book.

We strive to ensure the book runs smoothly, but we are not responsible for any temporary unavailability of the book due to factors outside our control. We hope you find the book enjoyable and appreciate your respect for the author's hard work.

CHAPTER 1 - INTRODUCTION

YOUR NEW FITNESS ALLY: WHY WALL PILATES WILL CHANGE YOUR LIFE

In the ever-evolving world of fitness, it seems there's always a new fad or trend emerging on the horizon. Some come and go as quickly as the seasons, while others manage to secure a lasting place in our workout routines. Enter Wall Pilates. This innovative and transformative approach to physical health isn't merely a passing trend—it's a revolution. When you think of Pilates, perhaps an image comes to mind of elegant studios filled with specialized equipment, like reformers and Cadillac machines. These traditional forms of Pilates are undoubtedly beneficial. But Wall Pilates breaks the mold, making the art of this renowned fitness routine more accessible than ever. It's time to understand why Wall Pilates is your new fitness ally and how it stands apart in the crowded fitness landscape.

The Genius Simplicity of Wall Pilates

The appeal of Wall Pilates stems from its straightforwardness. Rather than relying on expensive, bulky equipment or vast studio spaces, all you need is a sturdy wall. This not only makes it an incredibly cost-effective workout option but also ensures that it's a practice you can take anywhere—your home, office, or even while traveling. It's the democratization of fitness, ensuring that no matter your economic or spatial constraints, the power of Pilates remains within reach.

Unparalleled Customization

Traditional gym exercises or classes often follow a one-size-fits-all approach, which can be both frustrating and limiting. Wall Pilates shines in its adaptability. Whether you are an experienced athlete or just starting out on your fitness journey, Wall Pilates can be customized to meet your specific needs, tackle your challenges, and achieve your objectives. The wall provides feedback and resistance, allowing for micro-adjustments that cater to your specific strengths and areas of improvement. This personalization is rarely seen in other fitness regimens.

Beyond the Physical: The Mental Edge

Sure, in the next chapter, we'll delve deeper into the specific physical benefits of Wall Pilates. But let's not overlook the profound mental and emotional advantages. Engaging in Wall Pilates demands mindfulness—it's a meditative experience that fosters a deep connection between mind and body. This integration not only amplifies the physical results but also nurtures mental resilience, focus, and clarity. In a world fraught with distractions, the centeredness achieved through Wall Pilates is invaluable.

Why Choose Wall Pilates Over Other Sports?

1. **Economical & Space-Savvy**: Unlike other sports that require extensive gear or dedicated spaces, Wall Pilates is minimalist. You invest less but gain more in terms of health benefits.
2. **Low Impact, High Reward**: While high-impact sports can strain joints and muscles, Wall Pilates is gentler. This ensures a reduced risk of injuries while still delivering transformative results.
3. **Holistic Approach**: Beyond mere physical strength, Wall Pilates encourages posture perfection, mental fortitude, and emotional balance. Few sports can boast such a comprehensive impact.
4. **Flexibility in Routine**: Not feeling the full studio session today? No problem. Wall Pilates allows you to modify your routine based on energy levels, mood, or available time, making it more sustainable in the long run.

Stepping Into a New Era of Fitness

While sports like running, swimming, or traditional gym workouts have their merits, Wall Pilates introduces an unparalleled combination of flexibility, strength training, and mental conditioning. It's not about replacing these activities but enhancing your fitness repertoire.

The world of fitness is crowded, with countless activities vying for our attention. However, few offer the simplicity, effectiveness, and holistic benefits of Wall Pilates. As you delve deeper into this book, equipped with real photos to guide your exercises, you'll discover not just a series of movements but a transformative journey.

Choosing Wall Pilates isn't merely about adopting a new exercise routine. It's about embracing a lifestyle that prioritizes holistic well-being, anchored by a practice that's both timeless and innovative. Welcome to the next era of physical fitness. Welcome to Wall Pilates.

THE BENEFITS OF WALL PILATES FOR WOMEN

In today's fast-paced world, every woman seeks a fitness routine that not only caters to her health goals but also resonates with her unique body dynamics. Wall Pilates isn't just another exercise fad; it's an empowering practice steeped in understanding the nuances of the female form. From the ambitious professional to the dedicated mother, Wall Pilates is designed with the modern woman in mind, offering a harmonious blend of strength, flexibility, and balance. As we venture into this chapter, we will unravel the comprehensive advantages that this transformative workout brings to the table, setting the foundation for a healthier, stronger, and more confident you.

1. Targeted Muscle Engagement

Wall Pilates is precision in action, honing in on specific muscle groups to ensure maximum effectiveness.

- **Core**: Central to the Wall Pilates experience is the core. The powerhouse, spanning from the bottom of your ribs to your hips, is the epicenter of all movements in Wall Pilates. Regular engagement of this region diminishes belly fat, accentuates the abdominal muscles, and offers unparalleled support to the back. Moreover, a robust core aids in everyday activities, enhancing overall functional fitness and reducing the risk of injuries.

- **Glutes**: The promise of perky, firm glutes is no longer confined to grueling gym sessions. Wall Pilates offers a targeted approach. Using the wall as a source of resistance, the exercises designed for the glutes ensure they are consistently engaged, leading to improved lift and tone. Over time, this not only shapes the buttocks but also offers support to the lower back, reducing strain.

- **Legs**: The elegance of toned legs is a pursuit of many. Wall Pilates' diverse range of exercises engages everything from the hamstrings to the calves. The emphasis is on elongation and strength without adding bulk. This results in legs that are not just aesthetically pleasing but also powerful and less prone to fatigue.

2. Caloric Burn

While Wall Pilates may appear deceptively serene, it's a silent calorie torcher. A 1-hour session can incinerate between 180 to 270 calories. These figures, of course, vary based on age, weight, and overall exertion during the workout. However, there's a dual benefit here. Regular participation not only ensures calories are burned during the session but also leads to an increase in lean muscle mass. This heightened muscle profile revs up the resting metabolic rate, ensuring calorie burn even when at rest.

3. Improved Flexibility

In the realm of fitness, strength without flexibility is a recipe for disaster. Tight, rigid muscles are injury-prone. Wall Pilates offers the perfect blend of strength training with flexibility. As each move stretches the muscles, practitioners experience reduced stiffness, enhanced range of motion, and a marked reduction in muscle-related discomforts. Over time, this flexibility translates to better performance in other activities and a graceful ease in daily movements.

4. Enhanced Posture

Our modern lifestyles, dominated by screens, have given rise to the epidemic of poor posture. Wall Pilates is the antidote. Each exercise, when executed against the wall, becomes a lesson in alignment. The wall's flat surface acts as an immediate posture corrector, ensuring deviations are spotted and rectified. Continuous practice instills these postural corrections, leading to a naturally upright stance, minimized back issues, and even improved respiratory and digestive functions due to the optimal positioning of internal organs.

5. Tailored for Female Physiology

Wall Pilates is exceptionally beneficial for the unique physiology of women. Emphasis on the core inadvertently strengthens the pelvic floor—a critical muscle group for women. This hammock of muscles supports vital organs, aids in childbirth, and plays a pivotal role in bladder control and sexual health. Especially post-childbirth, Wall Pilates can be instrumental in regaining pelvic strength, combating postpartum issues like incontinence.

6. Stress Reduction

The symbiotic relationship between physical well-being and mental health is undeniable. Wall Pilates, with its rhythmic movements synchronized with deep breaths, offers a meditative respite. Each session becomes a sanctuary, allowing for the release of pent-up stress, tensions, and anxieties. Regular practitioners often report improved sleep patterns, better mood regulation, and a general sense of well-being.

7. Bone Health

For women, especially those approaching or undergoing menopause, bone health becomes paramount. Decreasing estrogen levels put them at a higher risk for osteoporosis. Wall Pilates, being a weight-bearing exercise where one pits their body weight against the wall, can be instrumental in maintaining, and sometimes even augmenting, bone density. This, consequently, lowers the risk of fractures, ensuring mobility and independence in the later years.

Conclusion

Wall Pilates, with its multi-pronged approach, addresses the gamut of women's fitness needs. Beyond aesthetics, it's a regimen rooted in health, strength, and holistic well-being. As you journey through these exercises, remember that each movement, each stretch, is a tribute to the incredible resilience and versatility of the female form. Embrace Wall Pilates, and let it be the cornerstone of your fitness journey.

PRECAUTIONS AND SAFETY TIPS

Wall Pilates, with its myriad of benefits, is more than just an exercise—it's a transformative journey. But like any journey, to ensure it's both fulfilling and safe, certain precautions are paramount. Here, we'll shed light on the most essential safety measures you should integrate into your Wall Pilates routine.

1. Always Start With a Warm-Up

Think of warming up as setting the stage for the main act. Before any Wall Pilates routine, it's vital to prepare the body with a 5-10 minute warm-up session. Not only does this increase blood flow, but it also enhances muscle elasticity and reduces the chances of strains. Opt for light aerobic exercises, like jumping jacks or high knees, and combine them with dynamic stretches targeting the major muscle groups. A proper warm-up will not only prime the body for the workout ahead but also improve overall performance.

2. Wear Appropriate Attire

The attire you choose can significantly impact the quality of your workout. With Wall Pilates, it's advised to wear form-fitting attire. This type of clothing allows you to see and correct your form while ensuring no fabric gets in the way of movements. Furthermore, breathable materials help regulate body temperature, preventing overheating. Lastly, avoid any clothing with zips or hard elements, as these could scratch or damage your wall.

3. Ensure Proper Footwear

Though traditional mat Pilates typically sees practitioners barefoot, Wall Pilates poses a slightly different scenario. Depending on your comfort level, you might opt for non-slip socks or even specialized Pilates shoes. The key is to ensure that whatever you wear offers a grip to prevent sliding, particularly when pushing off from or sliding down the wall.

4. Choose the Right Surface

The "wall" in Wall Pilates is as much a tool as it is a support, so its selection is critical. Ensure the wall you choose is sturdy, flat, and free from obstructions like wall hangings or decorations. A smooth, clean surface is essential for preventing injuries and ensuring a consistent workout experience. Moreover, the area should be spacious, permitting full range movements without any spatial restrictions.

5. Maintain Alignment

Alignment is the backbone of any Pilates form. The emphasis on a neutral spine in Wall Pilates means ensuring that the back is neither overly arched nor tucked. Proper alignment reduces stress on the spine, distributes weight effectively, and maximizes the benefits of each exercise. To self-check, use visual cues like shadows or reflections, or better yet, occasionally practice in front of a mirror.

6. Stay Hydrated

While Wall Pilates may not seem as intense as some other workouts, it's still a physically demanding activity. Hydration aids muscle contractions, joint flexibility, and temperature regulation. Make sure to have a water bottle nearby, and take little sips during your session to keep your hydration levels up. Remember, thirst is often a late indicator, so don't wait until you're thirsty to drink.

7. Listen to Your Body

The mantra "No pain, no gain" doesn't entirely apply here. While a mild discomfort or the feeling of muscles working is normal, sharp or persistent pain is a red flag. Every body is different, and what works for one might not for another. Modify exercises that feel uncomfortable, and if pain persists, consider consulting a physical therapist or expert.

8. Gradually Increase Intensity

Rome wasn't built in a day, and neither is the perfect physique. Begin with basic exercises to develop strength and familiarity. As you become more at ease, you can incorporate more demanding exercises or prolong the duration of your sessions. This gradual approach lowers the risk of injury and gives the body sufficient time to adapt and become stronger.

9. Keep Your Surroundings Clear

Your immediate environment plays a significant role in your safety. The area around the wall should be devoid of any tripping hazards. Ensure that mats are securely placed to prevent slipping, and always be aware of your surroundings, especially if you're in a shared space.

10. Post-Workout Care

The moments immediately after your workout are as crucial as the workout itself. Incorporate a relaxing phase featuring static stretches aimed at the muscles you've engaged. This aids in lactic acid dispersion, reducing muscle soreness. Furthermore, consider adding recovery tools like foam rollers or massage balls to help relax tight spots and enhance circulation.

Conclusion

Safety and effectiveness in Wall Pilates are two sides of the same coin. By taking these precautions to heart and regularly revisiting them, you set yourself up for a rewarding and injury-free Pilates journey. Remember, the essence of Pilates, whether on a mat or a wall, lies in controlled, mindful movements. Prioritize safety, and you'll find that the benefits naturally follow.

CHAPTER 2 - WALL PILATES FOUNDATIONS

BASIC PRINCIPLES OF PILATES

Pilates, over the decades, has been an integral part of the fitness lexicon. Its impact is vast, and its methodology profound. Joseph Pilates, the founder of this discipline, didn't merely concoct a series of exercises; he engineered a holistic system grounded in principles aimed at harmonizing the body and mind. As we approach the variant of Wall Pilates, a comprehensive understanding of these principles is not just beneficial but quintessential. They act as the compass, guiding each motion, ensuring the efficacy of every stretch, and setting the rhythm for every breath.

1. Centering

Often dubbed the 'Powerhouse', the center of the body plays a pivotal role in the realm of Pilates. This specific region spans from the lower ribs to the hip line, comprising the abdominal muscles, the lower back, hips, and the glutes. Every time a Pilates enthusiast embarks on an exercise, they're not just moving limbs but channeling energy from this central core. By persistently drawing attention to this zone, it becomes the nexus of all physical energy.

Technical Insight: In biomechanical terms, the powerhouse acts as the body's primary stabilizer. Engaging the core muscles not only enhances posture but also aids in motion transfer, allowing for efficient movement patterns. It's not just about chiseling the abs or achieving a desirable physique. It's about instilling functional strength, ensuring that each step we take and each movement we make is grounded in stability.

2. Concentration

Pilates is a symphony of mindfulness and movement. It isn't a mere physical endeavor; it's a dance where the mind leads and the body follows. Every twist, bend, and stretch in Pilates is accompanied by a conscious awareness, ensuring the movements are efficient, purposeful, and harmonious.

Technical Insight: From a neurological standpoint, concentration optimizes the neuromuscular pathways. As the brain becomes more attuned to the body's motions, there's a refined muscle activation, reducing the wastage of energy and maximizing the utilization of relevant muscle groups. This conscious engagement also aids in preventing injuries by ensuring that no muscle group is overstrained or overlooked.

3. Control

Where many fitness regimes rely on momentum, Pilates emphasizes controlled, mindful movements. There's a deliberateness to every action, ensuring that exercises are not driven by momentum but by muscular engagement. This approach not only guarantees that the targeted muscle groups are effectively activated but also significantly curbs the risk of undue strains or injuries.

Technical Insight: The beauty of controlled movements lies in their ability to enhance muscle fiber recruitment. As movements are decelerated and controlled, there's a greater emphasis on muscle engagement rather than momentum. This approach not only ensures a better workout intensity but also safeguards joints by preventing jerky, abrupt motions.

4. Precision

Pilates is not a race; it's a meticulous journey. It's not about the number of reps you perform, but the precision of each execution. The emphasis on precision ensures that every motion is optimized, every alignment is perfect, and every posture is correct.

Technical Insight: Precision plays a crucial role in biomechanics. Accurate movements ensure that the load is distributed correctly across the muscles and joints, minimizing the risk of wear and tear or overuse injuries. Moreover, precise movements lead to enhanced muscle memory, ensuring that over time, the body learns to move more efficiently, even outside the Pilates studio.

5. Breath

Breathing is the rhythmic backdrop to the Pilates melody. It's not a passive act but a dynamic component of the practice. By coordinating breath with movement, there's a synchronization of the internal and external, ensuring that the body is oxygenated optimally.

Technical Insight: Breathing has profound physiological implications. Deep, rhythmic breathing enhances oxygen uptake, ensuring that muscles receive the necessary fuel to function. Furthermore, exhaling during intense phases of an exercise can aid in better core engagement, amplifying the effectiveness of the workout.

6. Flow

Pilates is poetry in motion. There's an inherent grace, a fluidity that connects one movement to the next. This continuity ensures that the body remains engaged, muscles are consistently activated, and the session becomes a cohesive, holistic experience.

Technical Insight: From a physiological standpoint, continuous movement means muscles remain under tension for extended periods, enhancing muscular endurance. This constant engagement not only tones muscles but also heightens caloric expenditure, aiding in fat loss and body sculpting.

7. Flexibility

Pilates beautifully marries strength and flexibility. While the exercises are potent in toning and strengthening, they're equally effective in enhancing flexibility. Each stretch elongates the muscles, promotes joint health, and ensures a balanced, agile physique.

Technical Insight: A balance between strength and flexibility ensures that muscles are robust yet pliable. This harmony reduces the risk of injuries like strains or sprains. Furthermore, flexible muscles aid in better posture, ensuring that the spine remains neutral and the body remains agile.

Conclusion:

Understanding the principles of Pilates is akin to reading the notes before playing the music. They set the tone, the rhythm, and the essence of the practice. As we venture deeper into Wall Pilates in subsequent chapters, remember these principles as they form the bedrock of the discipline. Whether it's the traditional mat-based Pilates or the innovative Wall variant, these principles remain steadfast, guiding each of us towards a body that's not just aesthetically pleasing but functionally formidable.

POSTURAL ART: ALIGNMENT AND STABILITY

Amidst the rich tapestry of fitness disciplines, Wall Pilates stands out, not just for its transformative effects on the body, but for its meticulous attention to postural alignment and stability. Dubbed the "Postural Art," this discipline is more than a set of exercises—it's a dance of the spine, a ballet of balance, and a song of symmetry. As we peel back the layers of this art form, we discover the pillars of alignment and stability that are not just foundational but revolutionary in cultivating a body that's poised, powerful, and graceful.

1. The Essence of Alignment

Alignment, in Wall Pilates, isn't a mere buzzword. It's the lifeblood of the discipline. A body out of alignment is like a building with a skewed foundation—it may stand, but it's prone to early deterioration.

Anatomy of Alignment: The human body, when observed in the sagittal plane (from the side), displays a delicate curve—a forward curve in the cervical (neck) and lumbar (lower back) regions and a backward curve in the thoracic (mid-back) and sacral (pelvic) regions. Wall Pilates emphasizes maintaining these natural curves, ensuring the spine isn't hyperextended or overly flexed.

Technical Insight: From the base of the skull (occiput) to the tailbone (sacrum), alignment ensures even distribution of weight and pressure. Misalignment, even if subtle, can lead to muscle imbalances, uneven joint wear, and a cascade of potential injuries. In Wall Pilates, exercises are structured to reinforce and refine this alignment, using the wall as a tactile feedback mechanism.

2. The Symphony of Stability

In the universe of Wall Pilates, stability isn't stationary. It's dynamic, adapting to the ebb and flow of movement, ensuring the core remains engaged, the joints protected, and the movements fluid.

Foundation of Stability: Stability originates from the core—a robust belt of muscles that include the rectus abdominis, obliques, transversus abdominis, and the erector spinae. These muscles act as the body's natural corset, cinching the waist, supporting the spine, and serving as the launch pad for movement.

Technical Insight: While many fitness regimens focus on core strength, Wall Pilates extends the dialogue to core stability. Strength is about power, while stability is about control. Every exercise in Wall Pilates, from the most basic to the advanced, demands and develops both these facets, ensuring that as the core muscles sculpt and tone, they also learn to control and balance the body through a myriad of movements.

3. The Role of the Pelvis

Often overlooked in generic fitness routines, the pelvis is a pivotal player in postural alignment. Acting as the base of the spine, its orientation greatly affects the alignment of the vertebral column above it.

Pelvic Balance: The pelvis can tilt anteriorly (forward) or posteriorly (backward). An optimal position is a neutral pelvis, where it's neither tilted excessively forward nor backward, ensuring the natural lumbar curve is maintained.

Technical Insight: An anterior pelvic tilt, common due to sedentary lifestyles, can lead to lumbar hyperlordosis (excessive lower back curve) and a host of issues like lower back pain. Wall Pilates exercises often focus on pelvic stabilization, teaching practitioners to maintain a neutral pelvis, thereby optimizing lumbar spine health.

4. Wall Pilates: The Alignment Advantage

The brilliance of Wall Pilates in postural alignment lies in the wall itself. The wall serves as an immediate feedback tool, highlighting misalignments and aiding in correction.

The Wall as a Guide: As practitioners execute movements against the wall, any deviation from optimal alignment is instantly perceptible. This tangible feedback is invaluable in ingraining correct postural habits.

Technical Insight: With the wall acting as a constant reference point, there's less room for error. This not only makes Wall Pilates exceptionally effective in postural correction but also accelerates the learning curve, allowing practitioners to internalize and implement alignment principles faster.

5. Dynamic Stability in Movement

Wall Pilates is not about static holds—it's a dance of dynamic stability. While the wall assists in alignment, the real challenge lies in maintaining that alignment through movement.

The Dance of the Spine: From flexion to extension, from lateral bends to rotations, the spine moves in diverse planes. Wall Pilates exercises challenge this dynamism, demanding stability amidst motion.

Technical Insight: By emphasizing dynamic stability, Wall Pilates enhances proprioception—the body's sense of position in space. This not only aids in movement efficiency but also in injury prevention, as the body becomes adept at self-correction.

Conclusion:

Postural artistry in Wall Pilates is a journey from the surface to the profound depths of the body's architecture. Through meticulous attention to alignment and stability, it offers a route to a body that's not just sculpted but also harmoniously balanced. Whether you're a seasoned athlete or someone just stepping into the realm of fitness, understanding and embracing these principles will pave the way for a transformative journey—one where grace meets strength, and art meets anatomy.

BREATHING TECHNIQUES FOR AN EFFECTIVE WORKOUT

In the athletic world, the rhythm and depth of one's breath often determine the efficacy of a workout. Within the domain of Wall Pilates, breathing doesn't just fuel the body; it drives movement, supports the core, and deepens the mind-body connection. Let's journey into the world of breath, uncovering its significance, techniques, and strategies to harness its full potential during your Wall Pilates workouts.

1. The Rationale Behind Focused Breathing

Breathing seems innate, but when it comes to exercise, it turns into an art that requires mindfulness.

Physiological Impact: Every cell requires oxygen for optimal function. During Wall Pilates, the demand for oxygen surges. Proper breathing ensures a consistent oxygen supply, supporting muscle function and stamina. On other hand, superficial or irregular breathing can cause early tiredness and lessen the effectiveness of the exercise.

The Mind-Body Synergy: Focused breathing centers the mind, allowing for enhanced concentration on form and movement. It acts as a bridge, connecting mental intention with physical execution.

2. Lateral Breathing: The Pillar of Pilates

Lateral or thoracic breathing is the cornerstone of Pilates, including its wall-based variant.

Understanding Lateral Breathing: Unlike traditional vertical breathing, where the chest and shoulders rise, lateral breathing emphasizes expanding the ribcage sideways. This method allows the core to remain engaged during exercises, ensuring stability and alignment.

Technical Insight: To experience lateral breathing, place your hands at the sides of your ribcage. Inhale deeply, feeling the ribs push into your hands, expanding outwards. As you exhale, feel the ribs retracting back. The abdomen remains relatively still, keeping the core muscles engaged.

3. Coordinating Breath with Movement

Breath isn't just an accompaniment to movement in Wall Pilates; it's an integral component.

The Breath-Movement Dance: General thumb rule: Inhale during preparatory and lengthening movements, and exhale during exertion or when contracting muscles. For instance, if you're performing a wall slide, you'd inhale as you slide down, expanding and preparing the body. As you press back upwards, exhale and engage your core and leg muscles.

Technical Insight: Exhaling during exertion provides several benefits:

1. It helps engage the transverse abdominis, providing better core stability.
2. It allows for a more profound muscle contraction, heightening the exercise's effectiveness.
3. The forced exhalation can also help in extending the range of certain movements.

4. The Power of Paced Breathing

Paced breathing can elevate the efficacy of your Wall Pilates routines, helping manage exercise intensity.

The Science Behind Pacing: By consciously slowing down or speeding up the breath, one can influence heart rate and exercise intensity. Slow, deep breaths can help in recovery between intense exercise bursts, while quicker breaths can prepare and energize the body for upcoming exertions.

Technical Insight: During wall planks or holds, employing a slow, paced breathing technique can help in lengthening the hold time. The calming nature of slow breaths can mitigate the perception of exertion, allowing for extended durations.

5. Breathing Strategies for Enhanced Performance

Visualization: Mentally visualizing the path of the breath can enhance lung capacity utilization. Imagine the breath traveling from the nostrils, filling every lung corner, expanding the ribcage, and finally being expelled, pushing out every bit of stale air.

Audible Breath: There's a reason why certain exercise disciplines emphasize audible breathing. Hearing one's breath can act as a feedback mechanism, allowing instant corrections. If you notice your breathing becoming shallow or rapid, you can immediately adjust.

Breath Holds: While continuous breathing is emphasized, occasional breath holds (only when appropriate and safe) can strengthen the diaphragm and improve lung capacity. For instance, holding the breath momentarily during a core contraction and then exhaling forcefully can intensify the core engagement.

Conclusion:

The dance of Wall Pilates is as much about the ebb and flow of the breath as it is about the movements themselves. The symbiotic relationship between breathing and movement doesn't just amplify the workout's efficacy but also deepens the practitioner's connection to their body. As you journey through your Wall Pilates experience, let each inhalation bring awareness and preparation, and each exhalation drive intention and movement. The mastery of breath is, in many ways, the mastery of Wall Pilates itself.

CHAPTER 3 - EQUIPMENT AND PREPARATION

CREATING THE PERFECT CORNER: SELECTING AND PREPARING THE IDEAL SPACE

Every detail in a dedicated exercise space matters, right from the quality of air to the texture of the wall you're pressing against. Wall Pilates, being a unique discipline, requires a harmony of various elements. This chapter guides you through the intricate details of setting up that perfect space, ensuring you maximize the potential of every session.

1. The Art of Space Selection

Light and Ambience: Natural lighting not only reduces eye strain but also boosts serotonin levels, enhancing mood. Positioning your space close to a window can be rewarding. Morning rays, devoid of intense heat, can set a positive tone for the day. Meanwhile, late afternoon's golden hue can be incredibly soothing. If direct sunlight causes a glare, translucent curtains or blinds can filter and soften the light. For windowless rooms, ambient artificial lighting with adjustable brightness can mimic natural light to a degree. Opt for LED bulbs that mimic daylight tones.

Spaciousness: Space influences movement. Too constrained, and you risk incomplete motions; too vast, and it may lack the intimacy needed for focus. Ideally, a 6x6 feet space (1.8x1.8 meter) or larger is excellent. This permits stretches, extensions, and a range of movements. It's beneficial to visualize the exercises and routines you'll do, acting them out to see if the space feels right. Remember to consider ceiling height as well, especially for standing stretches.

Flooring Matters: The texture and material of your floor can directly impact your stability. Wooden floors, known for their grip and warmth, are top-tier choices. Vinyl floors, being water-resistant, are easy to clean after intense sessions where sweat might drop. Marble or tile can be tricky due to their slippery nature; hence, a high-grip mat or a textured carpet becomes necessary. Whatever your choice, the goal is to ensure you have a firm footing and are insulated from the cold.

2. Wall Integrity: Your Unsung Partner

Smooth Surface: Think of the wall as a silent partner in your Pilates journey. A smooth, consistent surface ensures uniformity in exercises. It's vital to inspect the wall for irregularities - protruding nails, chipped paint, or even patches of dampness. Address these issues by sanding down any rough spots, and if repainting, choose a matte finish to avoid unnecessary shine or reflection during sessions.

Wall Strength: The wall's robustness is paramount. Especially in homes with drywall installations, it's essential to ascertain that the wall can bear occasional pressure without any damage. For homes with traditional brick and mortar walls, this might be less of a concern. But regardless, checking for any signs of cracks or foundational weaknesses is pivotal.

Keep Distractions at Bay: Your wall should be a blank canvas, allowing you to focus purely on the exercise. Remove artwork, photo frames, or any decor. Switches and outlets, if within the area where you'll frequently interact with the wall, might need some adjusting. A consistent, distraction-free surface ensures you're mentally in the zone during each session.

3. The Anatomy of Essential Accessories

The Wall Mat: Much like the floor mat cushions your feet and body, a wall mat caters to your upper body. Depending on the texture of the wall, repeated leaning or pushing against it can cause discomfort. A wall mat, preferably made of foam or padded material, provides that buffer. It should be easy to clean, perhaps with a wipeable surface, ensuring hygiene is maintained.

Support Bars or Handles: These are game-changers for seasoned practitioners. Securely mounted bars or handles allow for advanced moves and provide stability for certain challenging exercises. Installation requires precision: the height, distance between bars, and their sturdiness need meticulous planning. Always hire a professional to fit these, ensuring they can bear weight and are fixed to wall studs for maximum safety.

Markers: Using removable and repositionable markers can help maintain the consistency of your poses. These markers serve as positioning guides for both hands and feet. Over time, as you gain confidence and muscle memory builds, the reliance on these markers may reduce. However, they're invaluable for beginners, ensuring exercises are done with precision right from the start.

4. Atmospheric Enhancements: Beyond the Physical

Sound: While Wall Pilates is a journey of inner connection, external elements like sound can influence it significantly. Soft instrumental tracks, nature-inspired sounds, or even rhythmic beats can set the pace and tone of the exercise. A quality speaker with clear sound output, preferably with Bluetooth connectivity, becomes an asset. Place it in a spot where it's easily accessible to change tracks or adjust volume.

Aroma: Our olfactory senses play a massive role in our mood. Utilizing a diffuser alongside essential oils can establish a mood. Lavender can be a wonderful calming agent, while peppermint or citrus oils can be uplifting and energizing. Always ensure the room doesn't become too overpowering with scent. A balance is key.

Ventilation: Breathing in fresh air can significantly improve the effectiveness of your exercises. A room that feels stuffy or stale can be demotivating. Ensure good ventilation. If exercising near a window, a mesh screen can keep out bugs while letting in the fresh air. An air purifier can be an excellent addition to rooms without windows.

5. Maintaining Your Space: The Ritual of Respect

Regular Cleaning: Cleanliness extends the life of your workout space. Post-session, it's prudent to wipe down areas where sweat might have splashed. A simple mixture of water and mild detergent, followed by a water-only wipe-down, keeps both wall and floor in prime condition. Always ensure the floor dries thoroughly to prevent slips in the next session.

Organizing Accessories: Dedicated storage solutions, be it shelves, drawers, or stylish storage boxes, can house your Pilates accessories. This organization ritual can be meditative. Arranging your gear post-session signals the brain about the session's conclusion, and setting up pre-session can mentally prepare you for the workout ahead.

Space Checks: Consistent inspections for wear and tear are non-negotiable. Check the wall for signs of moisture, chipping, or other damages. Similarly, inspect any installed handles or bars for any loosening. Immediate attention to these details guarantees safety.

Conclusion:

Your Wall Pilates space, curated with thought and care, becomes more than just a corner in your home. It embodies your commitment to health, balance, and inner strength. Crafting it with precision ensures every session is not just effective but also deeply fulfilling. This space, over time, will witness your transformation, bearing testament to your dedication and progress.

THE WALL PILATES KIT: RECOMMENDED TOOLS AND ACCESSORIES

When it comes to Wall Pilates, having the right equipment is not just about enhancing your workout but ensuring you execute each move with precision and safety. As the fitness world continues to innovate, there's a myriad of tools and accessories available to maximize your Wall Pilates experience. In this chapter, we'll break down the essential items for your Wall Pilates kit, shedding light on their function and offering recommendations for optimal usage.

1. The Pilates Wall Mat: Your Cushioned Companion

A quality Pilates wall mat is crucial. It provides a cushioned barrier between you and the wall, ensuring you can focus on your form without being distracted by discomfort.

- **Material Matters:** Opt for a mat made of dense foam or thick rubber. These materials offer a balance of cushioning and stability. They should possess the durability to endure the stress and wear from repeated exercises, thereby guaranteeing a long lifespan.
- **Size and Thickness:** A standard wall mat should measure around 24 inches (60cm) in width and 70 inches (178cm) in length. Regarding thickness, somewhere between 0.5 to 1 inch (1.25 to 2.55cm) is ideal, providing sufficient padding without compromising stability.

2. Resistance Bands: Adding Tension to the Mix

Resistance bands are versatile tools that can elevate the intensity of your Wall Pilates exercises. They enable you to engage your muscles differently, fostering strength and stamina.

- **Varieties:** Resistance bands come in various resistance levels – light, medium, heavy, and extra-heavy. Start with a medium band and adjust based on your strength and the specific exercise.
- **Material and Maintenance:** Latex or rubber bands are popular due to their elasticity and durability. To extend their lifespan, store them away from direct sunlight and avoid using oils or lotions before handling.

3. Pilates Ring (Magic Circle): The Multifunctional Marvel

The Pilates Ring, commonly known to as the "Magic Circle," is a flexible ring that offers resistance, challenging various muscle groups.

- **Usage Tips:** When using the ring, ensure it's appropriately positioned to avoid strain. It can be used between the thighs, hands, or even ankles, adding an element of resistance to standard Wall Pilates moves.
- **Selection Advice:** Look for a ring made of flexible plastic or rubber with padded handles. The diameter should be around 13 to 15 inches (33 to 38cm), fitting comfortably within most users' grasp.

4. Pilates Balls: Small But Mighty

These small, inflatable balls can be used in a variety of Wall Pilates exercises to improve balance, coordination, and muscle activation.

- **Sizing and Inflation:** Typically, these balls have a diameter of 7 to 9 inches (17.80 to 22.90cm). They should be inflated to a firmness where they can be slightly squeezed but not easily compressed.
- **Benefits:** Beyond balance and coordination, they can also provide tactile feedback, helping you become more aware of your body position and alignment during exercises.

5. Ankle Weights: Boosting the Challenge

Ankle weights add additional resistance to leg movements, amplifying the effort required and increasing the workout's benefits.

- **Weight and Adjustability:** Beginners should start with 1 to 2-pound (0.45 to 0.90kg) weights. Many ankle weights come with adjustable pockets, allowing you to customize the weight as you progress.
- **Comfort and Fit:** Ensure the weights have a secure yet comfortable strap. They should fit snugly around the

ankle without causing irritation or restricting circulation.

6. Wall Anchors: Safety First

While not exclusively a Pilates tool, wall anchors are essential for ensuring all wall-mounted equipment remains securely in place.

- **Installation:** It's crucial to install wall anchors into wall studs, not just the drywall. This guarantees the highest level of holding power. If you're uncertain about the installation, it's recommended to consult a specialist.
- **Types:** Depending on the wall type and the weight of the equipment, you might need toggle anchors, expansion anchors, or molly bolts.

In conclusion, assembling your Wall Pilates kit carefully is a crucial move towards ensuring your success. With the right tools at your disposal, each session will not only be more effective but also safer. As you expand your Pilates journey, these accessories will become trusted companions, aiding in your transformation. Remember, investing in quality now pays dividends in the benefits you reap later.

WARM-UP: PRELIMINARY EXERCISES

In the dynamic world of fitness, warming up isn't just a prologue to the main event; it's a fundamental chapter that sets the stage for what's to come. Before diving deep into the rigorous stretches and core-strengthening exercises of Wall Pilates, it's imperative to understand the importance of preliminary exercises. Just as an athlete doesn't directly jump onto the track without a proper warm-up, a Wall Pilates practitioner must ensure her body is primed for action.

Understanding the Role of Warm-Up

Warming up serves multiple purposes:

1. **Increasing Blood Flow:** Gentle exercises stimulate the circulatory system, gradually increasing the blood flow to your muscles. This is crucial for preparing the muscles for more intense activities, helping to prevent injury.
2. **Flexibility:** Preliminary stretches not only prepare the muscles for the movements ahead but also help in increasing overall flexibility. This flexibility will further assist in achieving the full range of motions in Wall Pilates exercises.
3. **Mental Preparation:** A warm-up serves not only the body but also the mind. These initial minutes help in mentally transitioning from the hustle and bustle of daily life to a focused exercise regimen.

Special Note on Imagery

As we transition into the exercise section of this book, we wish to share the rationale behind our choice of black and white imagery.

In this book, we've opted for monochromatic images over color. This deliberate decision is in line with our pledge to minimize our carbon emissions and advocate for eco-friendly practices. The production of color ink is associated with the use of chemicals and processes that are considerably more taxing on the environment compared to black and white ink. Moreover, printing in color consumes more energy, amplifying the environmental impact of this book.

By choosing black and white imagery, we aim to minimize these effects, making this book a more eco-conscious choice. Besides its green credentials, black and white photography holds a timeless aesthetic that encapsulates the essence of Wall Pilates - simplicity, elegance, and focus. It directs your attention to the form and technique of each exercise, free from the distractions of color.

This choice reflects our belief in mindful consumption and our responsibility toward promoting eco-friendly choices. As you delve into the exercises detailed in this book, the monochrome images echo the essence of Wall Pilates - creating a profound change through simple, thoughtful actions. Our hope is that this choice not only educates but also inspires our readers to adopt sustainable practices in their fitness journey and beyond.

The Wall Pilates Warm-Up Ritual

Let's delve into some effective preliminary exercises tailored for Wall Pilates:

1. **Wall-Assisted Neck Stretches:**

Technical Insight: Start by positioning yourself at a distance of an arm's length from the wall. Place your right hand on the wall, aligning it with you shoulder's height. Gently tilt your head to the left, stretching the right side of your neck. Hold for 20-25 seconds and repeat on the other side.

Benefits: This exercise provides a gentle stretch to the neck muscles, relieving any tension and preparing you for the forthcoming movements.

Duration & Repetitions: 3 sets x 30 seconds (for each side).

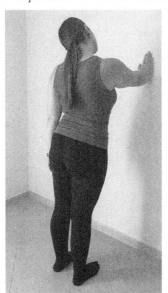 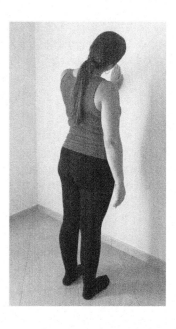

2. **Arm Circles with Wall Resistance:**

Technical Insight: Stand facing the wall, about six inches (15cm) away. Place both palms on the wall slightly higher than shoulder level. Now, move your hands in a circular motion (around the size of a dinner plate), letting the resistance of the wall challenge your muscles.

Benefits: This movement engages the deltoids and rotator cuff muscles, preparing them for more intensive activities.

Duration & Repetitions: 2 sets x 20 seconds (clockwise direction) + 2 sets x 20 seconds (counterclockwise direction).

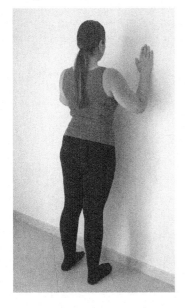 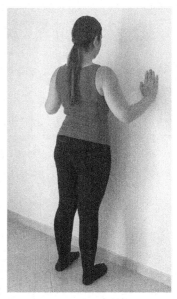

3. Wall Supported Leg Swings:

Technical Insight: Stand sideways to the wall, placing your hand on it for balance. Move the leg nearest to the wall forward and backward in a manner resembling a pendulum. After a few swings, switch to side-to-side leg swings. Switch legs after 30 seconds.

Benefits: This exercise warms up the hip flexors, hamstrings, and quads, all of which play pivotal roles in Wall Pilates.

Duration & Repetitions: 3 sets x 30 seconds for each leg.

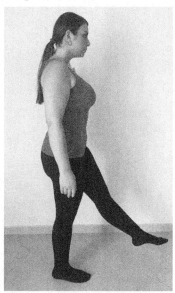 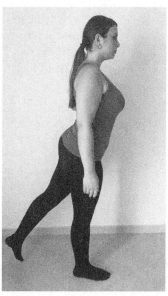

4. Wall Press and Chest Stretch:

Technical Insight: Position yourself at a distance of approximately two feet (60cm) from the wall, facing away from it. Reach back and place your palms on the wall, fingers pointing upward. Gradually deepen the stretch by pushing your chest outward and bringing your shoulder blades closer together.

Benefits: This warms up and stretches the chest muscles, ensuring they're flexible and ready for Wall Pilates postures.

Duration & Repetitions: 3 sets x 30 seconds.

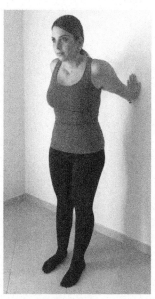

Warm-Up Duration and Intensity

An effective warm-up is typically between 10 to 15 minutes, ensuring all major muscle groups are activated. Remember, the aim isn't to tire yourself out but to prepare your body. The intensity should be moderate—enough to increase the heart rate and feel the stretch, but not so much that it leads to exhaustion.

COOLING DOWN: THE ESSENTIAL WIND-DOWN

As you ride the high from an invigorating session of Wall Pilates, it's tempting to call it a day and head straight for the shower. But, just as warming up preps your body for the workout ahead, cooling down is the crucial phase to help your body transition from intense activity back to its resting state. Think of it as a well-deserved "thank you" to your muscles for all the hard work.

The Significance of a Proper Cool Down

Cooling down isn't just a period of relaxation. It plays a pivotal role in:

1. **Easing muscle tension:** Stretching out worked muscles can minimize stiffness.
2. **Promoting recovery:** Boosting circulation can aid in flushing out lactic acid, which can cause muscle soreness.
3. **Re-establishing heart rate and blood pressure:** Gradually bringing down your heart rate helps avoid dizziness or fainting.

Cool Down Exercises Post Wall Pilates

- **Wall-Touch Forward Bend with Pulsations**
  1. Stand facing the wall.
  2. Pivot from your hips and lean forward until your upper body is level with the ground.
  3. Stretch out your arms and press your hand palms directly onto the wall.
  4. While keeping your arms firm and palms pressed to the wall, pulse your upper body gently downwards, getting a deeper stretch in the back and hamstrings. Perform these pulsations for 20-30 seconds, breathing steadily throughout.

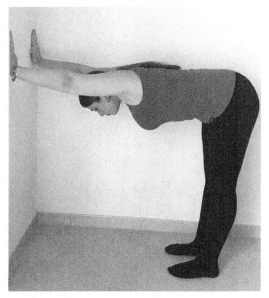

- **Wall Chest Opener**
  1. Stand side-on to the wall.
  2. Extend the arm nearest to the wall and position your palm against it.
  3. Gradually turn your body away from the wall, experiencing a stretch across your chest and the front of your shoulder. Maintain this position for 20-30 seconds and then do the same on the opposite side.

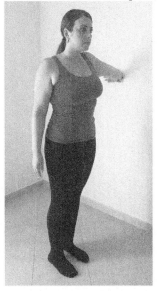
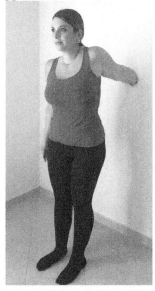

- **Quad Stretch with Wall Support**
  1. Face the wall and place both hands on it.
  2. Bend one knee, bringing the heel towards your glutes.
  3. Hold your ankle with the free hand. Keep your knees close together and push your hips forward to feel the stretch down the front of your thigh. Hold for a duration of 20 to 30 seconds, afterward change to the other leg.

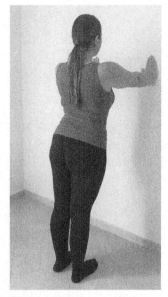 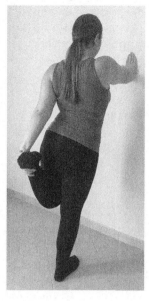

- **Deep Breathing**
  1. Stand or sit comfortably.
  2. Inhale deeply via your nose, allowing your abdomen to broaden.
  3. Exhale slowly through your mouth, focusing on emptying your lungs completely.
  4. Perform this action 5 to 10 times, letting your body sink into a deeper relaxation with every breath out.

Consistency is Key

Having a regular cool-down routine can markedly influence your overall fitness progress. It aids in preventing injuries, reducing muscle soreness, and providing a moment of calm reflection after the dynamism of your workout.

Take these moments to congratulate yourself. Every stretch, every breath taken post-workout is a testament to your commitment. As you gradually ease your body back to its resting pace, you're not just wrapping up a session — you're setting the stage for your next one, ensuring that you return to the wall rejuvenated and ready.

So, next time you're tempted to skip the cool-down, remember: this is your moment to honor your body's hard work, promote recovery, and pave the way for your next Wall Pilates session.

CHAPTER 4 - BASIC EXERCISES

WALL-POWERED PLANK REACH

Total Time: 5 minutes

Equipment Needed:
- A sturdy wall
- Exercise mat (optional for comfort)

Procedure:
1. Begin by facing away from the wall. The distance from the wall should be approximately 2 feet (0.6 meters). This guarantees your sufficient room to maneuver without hindrance. Stand tall with your feet hip-width apart.
2. Slowly lean forward, placing your hands onto the wall. Ensure your hands are spread as wide as your shoulder and aligned right beneath them for balance. Your body ought to create a slanted line stretching from your heels all the way to your head.
3. As you find stability in this inclined plank position, actively engage your core muscles. Press the balls of your feet into the ground, ensuring your legs remain straight and strong. This is your starting position.
4. Maintaining your plank alignment, slowly lift your right hand off the wall. Extend your arm upward toward the ceiling, reaching as high as possible without rotating your torso. Your body weight might shift, but the challenge is to keep the hips and shoulders squared to the wall.
5. After reaching out, slowly place your right hand back on the wall to regain your two-handed support. Then repeat the reaching motion with your left arm.
6. Throughout the exercise, ensure you're taking deep and controlled breaths. Exhale as you lift and reach out with your arm, and inhale as you return your hand to the wall.

Repetitions and Rest:
- 3 sets x 10 reps (per arm)
- Recovery: 10 seconds between sets

Advanced Variation: For those looking to enhance the challenge, try this on your toes! Rather than keeping your feet flat, elevate your eels and maintain balance on the front part of your feet as you execute the Wall-Powered Plank Reach. This adjustment requires extra calf strength and increased core stability, making the exercise more demanding.

STEP 1

STEP 2

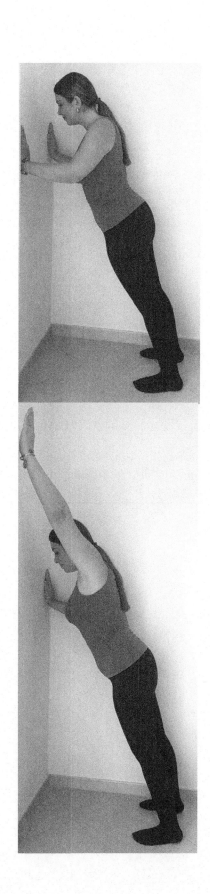

GLUTE BRIDGE WALL PRESS

Total Time: 5 minutes

Equipment Needed:
- A sturdy wall
- Exercise mat (for added comfort)

Procedure:
1. Start by positioning yourself on the exercise mat with your back flat on it, facing the ceiling. Arrange your legs so that your feet are pressed flat against the wall with your knees forming a 90-degree angle. The distance from the wall should be about 1 to 1.5 feet (0.3 to 0.45 meters).
2. Position your arms along your sides, with palms turned downwards. This provides additional stability during the exercise.
3. Engage your core and press your feet into the wall. While performing this action, elevate your hips from the floor, contracting the gluteal muscles when they reach the highest point. Your body should align straight from your shoulders down to your ankles.
4. While keeping the hips elevated, press your feet harder into the wall. This engages the hamstrings and glutes even further. Maintain this stance for several seconds to optimize muscle activation.
5. Gently bring your hips down to the initial position, making sure to execute a controlled movement for effective engagement of the core and glutes.

Repetitions and Rest:
- 3 sets x 12 reps
- Recovery: 15 seconds between sets

Advanced Variation: To intensify the exercise, once the hips are elevated and you're pressing your feet into the wall, lift one foot off the wall, extending it out straight. This not only challenges your glutes and hamstrings but also engages the core for added balance. Perform the required number of repetitions and then switch to the other foot.

STEP 1

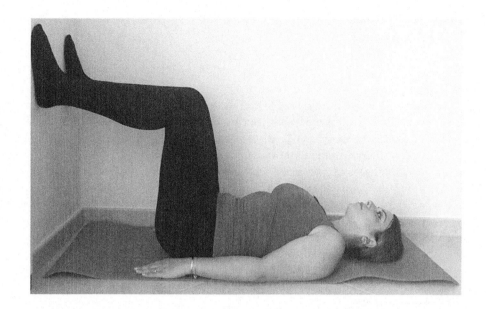

STEP 2

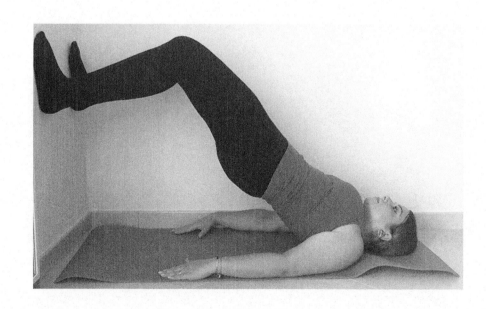

STANDING WALL LEG LIFTS

Total Time: 7 minutes

Equipment Needed:
- A sturdy wall
- Exercise mat (optional for comfort)

Procedure:
1. Begin by standing side-on to the wall, about 6 inches (16 cm) away. Your feet should be positioned at a width equivalent to your hips, with your inside foot (the one nearest to the wall) placed a bit ahead.
2. Extend your inside arm and place your palm flat against the wall for stability. Your hand should be at shoulder height, fingers pointing upwards.
3. Ensure that your back is straight, core engaged, and your head is aligned with your spine.
4. Slowly lift your outside leg (the one farthest from the wall) to the side, keeping the leg straight. Elevate the leg to a height where you can maintain control and form, typically no higher than hip height. Then, with control, lower the leg back down without allowing it to touch the ground. This completes one movement.
5. During the lifting and lowering action, keep your foot flexed (toes pointing forward, not up) and ensure the movement is powered by your hip muscles, not momentum.
6. After completing the set for one side, turn around and repeat the procedure with the opposite leg and arm.

Repetitions and Rest:
- 3 sets x 12 reps
- Recovery: 15 seconds between sets

Advanced Variation: To intensify the workout, add ankle weights to your lifting leg. Begin with a manageable weight and incrementally increase it as your strength gets better. Ensure you maintain proper form and avoid any jerky or swinging motions.

STEP 1

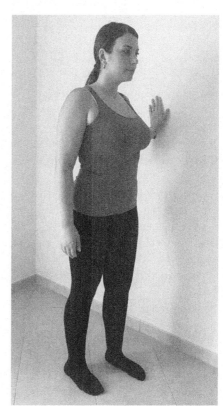

STEP 2

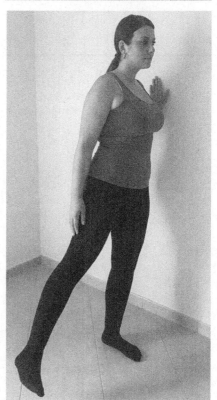

CORE-ENGAGING WALL SQUAT

Total Time: 8 minutes

Equipment Needed:
- A sturdy wall
- Exercise mat (optional for added comfort)

Procedure:
1. Start by positioning yourself with your back against the wall. The distance from your feet to the wall should be about 12 to 14 inches (30 to 35 centimeters), ensuring you have enough space to lower your body into a squat position.
2. Plant your feet shoulder-width apart, firmly on the ground. Your toes should point slightly outward.
3. Keep your back flat against the wall and engage your core muscles. This will act as your stabilizing force throughout the exercise.
4. Gradually glide your back down along the wall, flexing your knees but keeping your feet firmly on the ground. Descend until your thighs form a horizontal line with the floor, mirroring a sitting posture. Ensure that your knees are positioned right above your ankles and do not extend past your toes.
5. As you hold the squat position, draw your navel towards your spine to engage the core muscles further. Maintain a firm core throughout the motion.
6. Press down on your heels, extend your knees, and glide your back upward along the wall to get back to the initial position.

Repetitions and Rest:
- 3 sets x 15 reps
- Recovery: 20 seconds between sets

Advanced Variation: For a more challenging workout, hold a dumbbell in each hand by your sides while performing the squat. Ensure that the weight does not compromise your form. If using weights, make sure they're of an appropriate weight that doesn't strain your back or knees. As your strength progresses, you can gradually increase the weight.

STEP 1

STEP 2

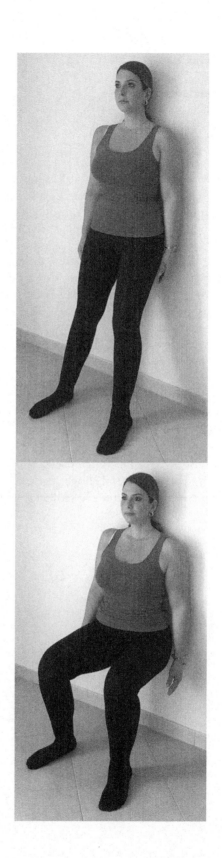

WALL SLIDE SHOULDER ELEVATIONS

Total Time: 5 minutes

Equipment Needed:
- A sturdy wall
- Exercise mat (for added comfort)

Procedure:
1. Begin by standing facing the wall, approximately 12 inches (30 centimeters) away. Position your feet so they're aligned with your hips, and maintain a straight posture.
2. Reach your arms out in front of you and press your palms firmly against the wall at the level of your shoulders, spreading your fingers out to enhance stability.
3. Activate your abdominal muscles and make sure your back remains straight. Your nose and toes should be facing the wall, and heels firmly planted on the floor.
4. Begin by slowly sliding your hands upwards along the wall, keeping full palm contact. Aim to raise your arms as high as possible without any part of your palm or fingers losing contact with the wall.
5. As you slide your hands up, elevate your shoulders towards your ears, ensuring you maintain a straight back and an engaged core.
6. Gradually slide your hands back down the wall to the initial position, lowering your shoulders away from your ears as you do so.

Repetitions and Rest:
- 3 sets x 10 reps
- Recovery: 15 seconds between sets

Advanced Variation: To intensify the exercise, hold a light resistance band (with both ends) between your hands while performing the movement. The band should be taut but not strained. As you slide your arms up the wall, stretch the band slightly, maintaining constant tension. This will engage the shoulder muscles more and provide added resistance throughout the movement.

STEP 1

STEP 2

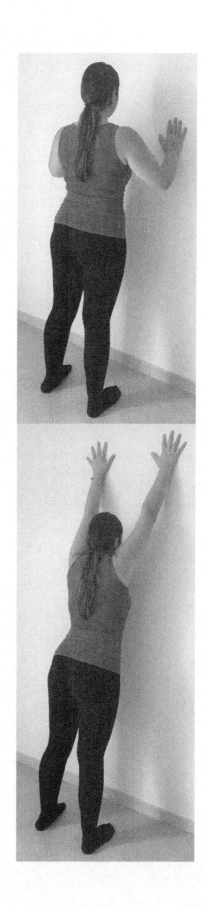

WALL-ASSISTED LEG CIRCLES

Total Time: 6 minutes

Equipment Needed:
- A sturdy wall
- Exercise mat

Procedure:
1. You can start by positioning yourself on the exercise mat, ensuring your back is flat on the ground. Set both your feet against the wall, ensuring your knees form a right angle. Your hips should be roughly 18 inches (45 centimeters) away from the wall.
2. Stretch your right leg straight upward toward the ceiling, while pointing your toes.
3. Start making controlled circular movements in the air with your right foot. Ensure the movement is driven from the hip joint and not the knee, keeping the rest of your body still and core engaged. The diameter of the circles should be roughly the same as that basketball.
4. After completing the set for one leg, bring the right foot back to the wall and extend the left leg to repeat the circles.
5. Ensure your spine remains in neutral alignment throughout the exercise. Avoid arching your back by keeping the core muscles engaged and pressing the lower back gently into the mat.

Repetitions and Rest:
- 3 sets x 10 circles (each direction) for each leg
- Recovery: 20 seconds between sets

Advanced Variation: To make the exercise more challenging, move your hips closer to the wall, reducing the angle of the bent knee (less than 90 degrees). This will require greater stability and control from your core as you draw the circles with your leg. Remember to keep the motion smooth and maintain a steady breathing pattern.

STEP 1

STEP 2

STANDING WALL TWIST

Total Time: 5 minutes

Equipment Needed:
- A sturdy wall

Procedure:
1. Position yourself so that your right side is towards the wall, with your feet spaced the width of your hips.
2. With arms bent at shoulder level, ensure your palms are oriented forward. Your right hand should lightly touch the wall.
3. Keeping your hips and feet fixed forward, begin to rotate your torso to the left. Allow your right hand to slide on the wall as you twist, and your left hand to move backward, following the twist. Your head and eyes should follow the movement of your left hand.
4. Rotate your torso as far to the left as comfortably possible, feeling a stretch in your oblique muscles. Maintain this stance for a few seconds before gently reverting to the initial position.
5. Upon finishing the set, rotate so your left side is oriented towards the wall, and perform the exercise again, this time twisting to the right

Repetitions and Rest:
- 3 sets x 10 twists (for each side)
- Recovery: 15 seconds between sets

Advanced Variation: To increase the intensity of the exercise, hold a lightweight (like a dumbbell or kettlebell) in both hands as you twist. As you rotate your torso, the weight should move in a horizontal arc, adding resistance to the twist and further engaging your core. Ensure the movement remains controlled to avoid any strain or injury.

STEP 1

STEP 2

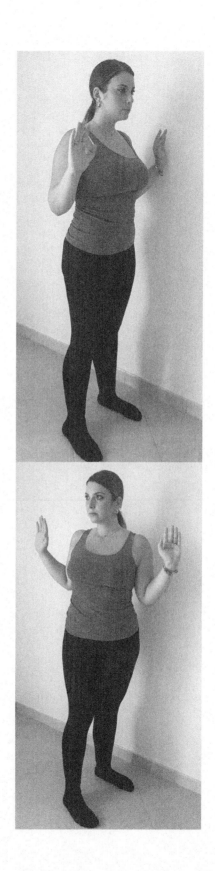

SINGLE-LEG WALL PUSH-OFF

Total Time: 10 minutes

Equipment Needed:
- Wall
- Exercise mat (optional for added comfort)

Procedure:
1. Begin by standing approximately 2 feet (60 cm) away from the wall, facing it directly.
2. Position both of your hands flat on the wall, with a distance a bit more than the width of your shoulders between them.
3. Engage your core and keep your back straight throughout the exercise.
4. Shift your body's balance onto your right foot while raising your left foot from the surface. Maintain balance and stability by pressing through your right heel and engaging your glutes and quadriceps.
5. Maintain control as you flex your elbows and incline your upper torso toward the wall, mimicking a push-up. Keep your right firmly planted on the ground while your left leg remains in a suspended position.
6. Propel yourself away from the wall by straightening your arms, returning to the initial stance. Ensure that you're using your chest and arm muscles to generate the force, and not solely pushing off with your foot.
7. Carry out the required amount of iterations before transitioning to the opposite leg.

Repetitions and Rest:
- 10 sets x 3 reps (for each leg)
- Recovery: 15 seconds between sets

Advanced Variation: To intensify the workout, after pushing off from the wall, add a single-leg hop on the standing foot while the other foot remains lifted. This not only strengthens the muscles but also enhances balance and coordination. Remember to land softly with a slight bend in the knee to reduce impact.

STEP 1

STEP 2

CHAPTER 5 - CORE STRENGTHENING EXERCISES

WALL MOUNTAIN CLIMBERS

Total Time: 5 minutes

Equipment Needed:
- Exercise mat (optional for added comfort)

Procedure:
1. Begin by positioning yourself into a plank position, facing away from the wall. Place your hands solidly on the floor, aligned directly below your shoulders. Ensure that there's a straight alignment from your head to your heels.
2. Position your feet against the wall, pointing your toes downward. Your body should form an incline with the floor.
3. Engaging your core, draw one knee toward your chest as you would in a regular mountain climber. As you do this, push the opposite foot firmly against the wall for stability.
4. Return the foot to the wall and quickly switch legs, pulling the other knee to your chest.
5. Continue alternating legs in a fast-paced manner, mimicking a climbing motion. Keep your spine aligned and maintain a tight core during the workout.

For safety: Ensure you're positioned at a distance where you can comfortably place your feet against the wall and can easily perform the climbing motion without straining your back.

Repetitions and Rest:
- 4 sets x 45 seconds
- Recovery: 30 seconds between sets

Advanced Variation: For those looking to up the ante, add a twist to the movement: as you bring one knee forward, twist your waist, aiming the knee toward the opposite elbow. This not only challenges the rectus abdominis but also the obliques, ensuring an all-encompassing core workout.

STEP 1

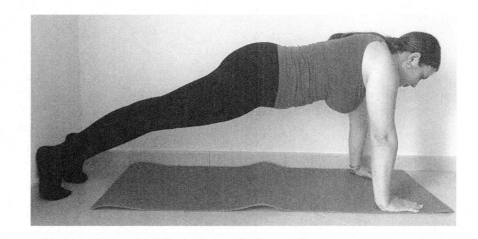

STEP 2

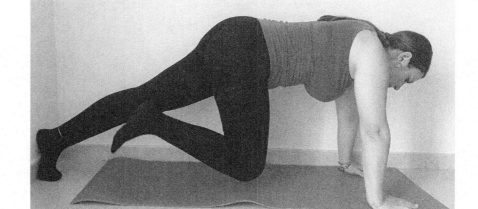

ISOMETRIC WALL PLANK HOLD

Total Time: 5 minutes

Equipment Needed:
- Exercise mat (optional)

Procedure:
1. Begin by standing approximately 2 feet (60 centimeters) away from a sturdy wall, facing towards from it.
2. Lean towards the wall and position your hands flat against it. Ensure your hands are spread as wide as your shoulders, with your wrists aligned with them.
3. Step your feet back, one at a time, until you're in a slanted plank position with your body forming a straight line from your head to your heels. The balls of your feet should be the only part touching the ground.
4. Engage your core, ensuring your hips don't sag or pike upwards. Your body should maintain a straight and stiff posture for the entire length of the exercise.
5. Maintain a neutral neck by gazing down at the ground, a few inches in front of your fingertips.
6. Hold this position, keeping your muscles engaged and breathing evenly.

Repetitions and Rest:
- 3 sets x 60 seconds hold
- Recovery: 30 seconds between sets

Advanced Variation: For a more challenging variation, after assuming the wall plank position, lift one leg off the ground, keeping it straight and aligned with your body. This will engage your core even more, as you'll be stabilizing with a single leg. Alternate legs with each repetition.

STEP 1

STEP 2

STEP 3

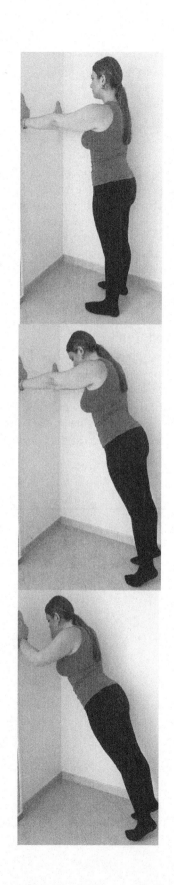

WALL LEG RAISES

Total Time: 8 minutes

Equipment Needed:
- Exercise mat

Procedure:
1. Begin by standing approximately 1 foot (30 centimeters) away from a sturdy wall, with your back against it.
2. Position your feet hip-width apart and press your lower back flat against the wall, eliminating any gap. This is crucial for spinal safety and to ensure maximum core engagement.
3. Place your arms by your sides with palms facing inwards, or on your hips for added balance.
4. Keeping your left foot firmly on the ground, slowly raise your right leg straight up in front of you, keeping the knee locked. Lift as high as your flexibility allows, ideally reaching a point where your leg is parallel to the floor.
5. Maintain engagement of your core muscles during the entire motion, making sure your back stays pressed flat against the wall.
6. Gently bring down the right leg and do the same action with the left one.

Repetitions and Rest:
- 3 sets x 10 reps (5 on each leg)
- Recovery: 30 seconds between sets

Advanced Variation: For an intensified challenge, after raising your leg to its peak height, add small pulses upwards, lifting and lowering the leg by a few inches for 5 additional counts before bringing the leg down completely. This will further activate the hip flexors and deepen the engagement of the core muscles.

STEP 1

STEP 2

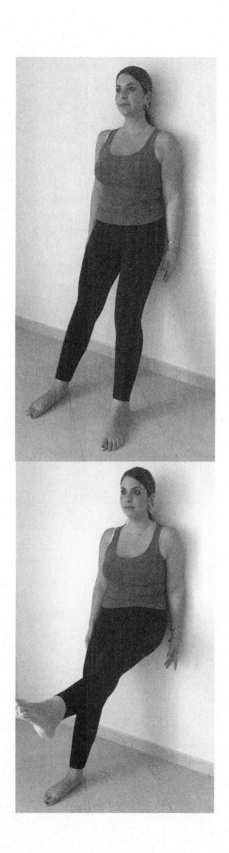

WALL OBLIQUE CRUNCHES

Total Time: 10 minutes

Equipment Needed:
- Exercise mat

Procedure:
1. Begin by standing sideways to a sturdy wall. For starting with the right oblique, your left side should be closest to the wall.
2. Stand approximately 1 foot (30 centimeters) away from the wall to give your body enough space to move.
3. Position your feet as wide as your shoulders and make sure they remain stable on the floor during the workout.
4. Extend your left arm straight above your head and place the back of your hand against the wall. This will be your stabilizing point.
5. While you breathe out, tighten your core and obliques, then raise your right knee, trying to touch your left elbow and right knee together. Make sure you're moving from the waist and not just the arms or legs.
6. Breathe in as you gradually go back to the initial position.
7. Repeat the motion for the desired repetitions, then switch to the other side, with your left side closest to the wall.

Repetitions and Rest:
- 3 sets x 12 reps (6 on each side)
- Recovery: 20 seconds between sets

Advanced Variation: To further challenge your obliques, after bringing your elbow and knee together, hold the crunch position and pulse for 3 counts before returning to the starting position. The pulses should be small and controlled, deepening the contraction in the oblique muscles with each pulse.

STEP 1

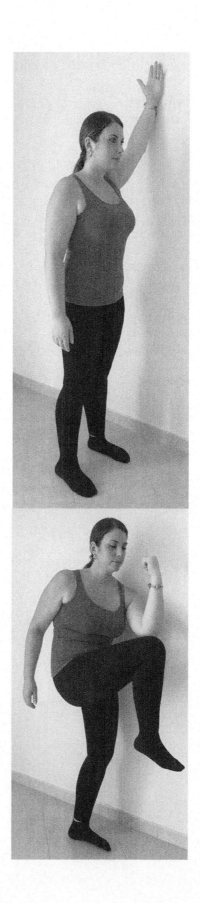

STEP 2

VERTICAL WALL SIT & TWIST

Total Time: 8 minutes

Equipment Needed:
- Exercise mat (optional)

Procedure:
1. Begin by standing approximately 2 feet (60 cm) away from the wall, with your back facing it.
2. Lean back to place your entire back against the wall, ensuring that your head, shoulders, and lower back maintain contact.
3. Descend along the wall by flexing your knees until they achieve a right angle. Make sure your knees are positioned directly over your ankles. Your thighs should be parallel to the ground, effectively getting into a "wall sit" position.
4. Stretch your arms forward, so they are level with the floor, with your hands joined together.
5. While exhaling, activate your core muscles. Gently twist your torso to the right side, aiming to bring both hands as close as possible to the wall on your right. Your right arm will move backward during this twist, but keep your back in contact with the wall.
6. Inhale as you return to the center.
7. Repeat the twist on the left side.
8. Ensure that during each twist, your hips and lower body remain stationary and only your upper body moves.

Repetitions and Rest:
- 5 sets x 4 reps (right and left twists count as one rep)
- Recovery: 15 seconds between sets

Advanced Variation: To intensify this exercise, hold a lightweight (like a dumbbell or a water bottle) in your hands as you perform the twist. This adds resistance to the movement, challenging your obliques even further. Remember to keep the movement controlled and avoid jerking or using momentum.

STEP 1-2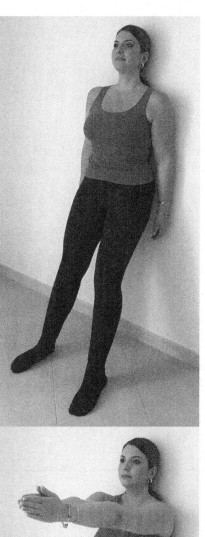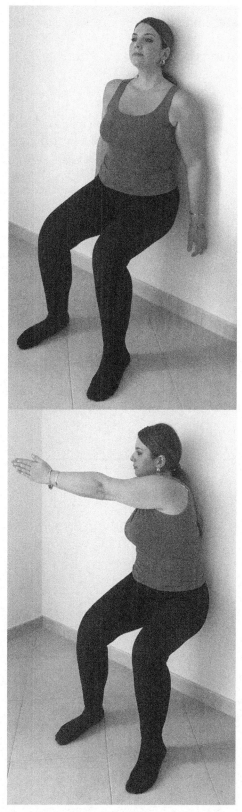

STEP 3-4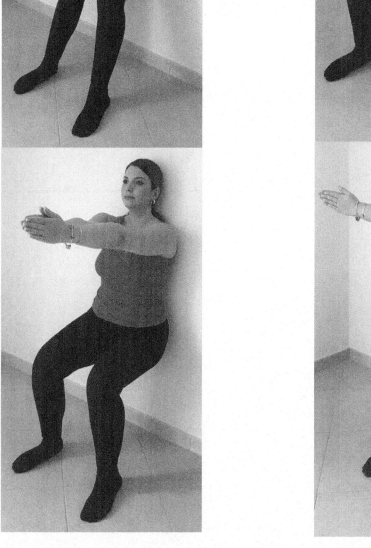

WALL DEAD BUG

Total Time: 10 minutes

Equipment Needed:
- Exercise mat

Procedure:
1. Position the exercise mat so that it forms a right angle with the wall. Lay down on the mat on your back, ensuring your head is pointed away from the wall and your arms are stretched straight up towards the ceiling.
2. Raise both of your legs and rest your feet against the wall, keeping your knees bent at a right angle.
3. As you press your left foot firmly against the wall, extend your right leg straight out, hovering just above the ground, while simultaneously lowering your left arm back towards the floor above your head.
4. Gently bring your right leg and left arm back to their initial positions.
5. Now, press your right foot against the wall, extend your left leg out while lowering your right arm in the same manner.
6. Throughout the exercise, ensure your lower back remains flat against the mat, and keep your head and upper back slightly lifted off the ground to further engage the core. Activate your core muscles to attain stability, focusing on the deep core muscles.

Repetitions and Rest:
- 3 sets x 12 reps (on each side)
- Recovery: 45 seconds between sets

Advanced Variation: To increase the challenge, introduce small hand weights for the moving arm, thus demanding more stability and engagement from the core muscles during each repetition.

STEP 1

STEP 2

STEP 3

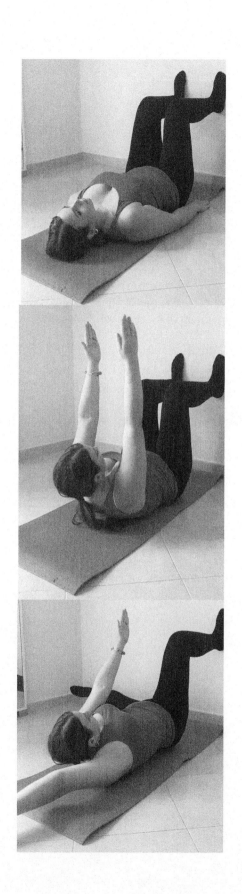

WALL DEAD BUG WITH ARM SLIDE

Total Time: 11 minutes

Equipment Needed:
- Exercise mat

Procedure:
1. Start by lying flat on your back on the exercise mat, positioning yourself perpendicular to the wall. Check that your head, shoulders, and lower back are solidly in contact with the mat.
2. Lift your legs and place your feet flat on the wall, with your knees bent at a 90-degree angle.
3. Extend your arms straight up towards the ceiling, fingers pointing upwards.
4. Engage your core. Keeping your lower back pressed firmly to the mat and your head and upper back lifted, begin with two movements. First, slowly slide your left hand upwards. Simultaneously, extend your right leg straight out, allowing it to hover just above the ground.
5. Return to the starting position.
6. Repeat the movement, this time sliding your right hand upwards while extending your left leg.
7. Continue to alternate sides for the duration of the exercise.

Repetitions and Rest:
- 3 sets x 12 reps (on each side)
- Recovery: 15 seconds between sets

Advanced Variation: To make this exercise more challenging, instead of sliding the hand upwards, push the hand into the wall while maintaining the slide. This will create resistance and further engage the core muscles.

STEP 1

STEP 2

STEP 3

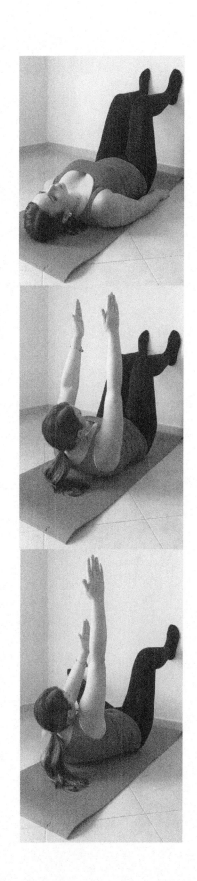

HIGH WALL KNEE TUCKS (INVERTED)

Total Time: 6 minutes

Equipment Needed:
- Exercise mat

Procedure:
1. Place your exercise mat perpendicular and close to the wall, ensuring there's enough clear space around you.
2. Your body should maintain a straight alignment from head to heels.
3. Extend your arms upwards and bend them at the elbows, positioning your hands by your ears.
4. Engage your core muscles, drawing your navel in towards your spine.
5. Employing the strength of your core, draw your knees towards your chest, raising them off the mat.
6. Stretch your legs out once more and revert to the initial position, halting just before they make contact with the ground. Maintain control throughout the motion, ensuring your legs don't drop abruptly.
7. Throughout the exercise, ensure consistent breathing: inhale as you extend your legs and exhale as you tuck your knees.

Repetitions and Rest:
- 3 sets x 15 reps
- Recovery: 30 seconds between sets.

Advanced Variation: For added challenge, once you've tucked your knees towards your chest, extend your legs upwards towards the ceiling, straightening them fully. Hold for a beat before returning to the initial position. This will further engage your core and intensify the abdominal workout.

STEP 1

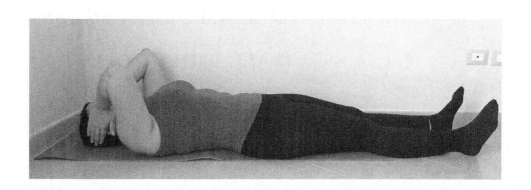

STEP 2

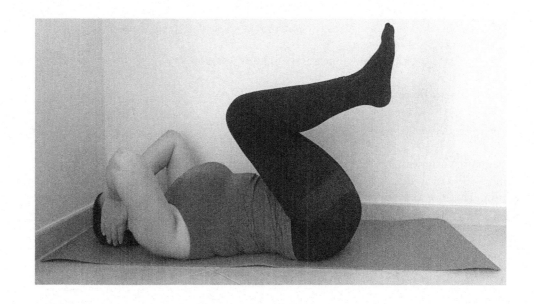

STEP 3

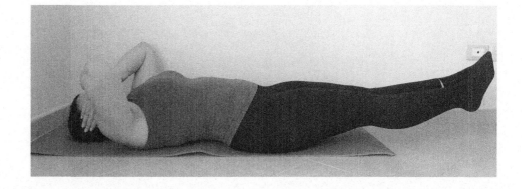

CHAPTER 6 - EXERCISES FOR LEGS AND GLUTES

WALL SQUAT HOLDS

Total Time: 6 minutes

Equipment Needed:
- None

Procedure:
1. Position yourself with your back touching a wall. Your feet should be positioned about 2 feet (60 cm) away from the wall and shoulder-width apart.
2. Begin by slowly sliding your back down the wall, bending your knees as if you're going to sit down in a chair. Your knees ought to align directly over your ankles, forming a right angle. Make sure your thighs are level with the floor.
3. Push your lower back against the wall. Maintain a relaxed position in your shoulders and prevent them from curling forward. Your hands can either be placed at your sides or resting on your thighs, but ensure they're not providing assistance.
4. Engage your core and glutes, and hold this position.

Repetitions and Rest:
- 5 sets x 60 seconds holds
- Recovery: 20 seconds between sets.

Advanced Variation: To challenge yourself further, try the Single-Leg Wall Squat Hold. Adhere to the same procedure, but when you reach the squat position, raise one leg off the ground while keeping it straight. Switch legs with every repetition. This not only intensifies the workout for the leg still on the ground but also engages your core more as you balance.

STEP 1

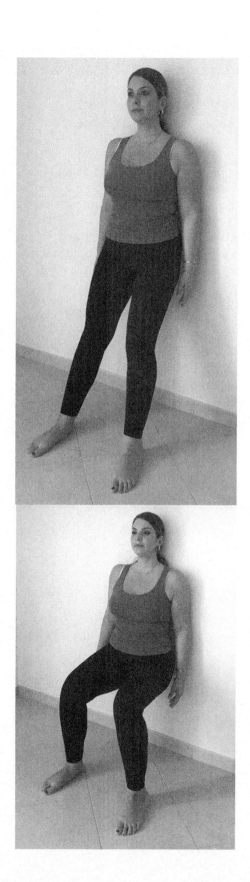

STEP 2

ELEVATED WALL LUNGES

Total Time: 8 minutes

Equipment Needed:
- None

Procedure:
1. Begin by positioning yourself approximately 3 feet (90 cm) away from the wall, with your back facing towards it.
2. Place your hands on your hips and ensure your feet are hip-width apart.
3. Take a step forward with your right foot, ensuring that your heel is firmly planted on the ground.
4. Elevate your left foot behind you and place the ball of that foot against the wall, creating an angle.
5. Lower your body towards the ground by bending both knees. Strive to have your right thigh parallel to the ground, while your left knee points downward, barely above the floor.
6. To return to the initial position, press down on your right heel, then alternate legs.

Repetitions and Rest:
- 4 sets x 10 lunges (5 per leg)
- Recovery: 30 seconds between sets.

Advanced Variation: For a more intense workout, try the Elevated Wall Lunge Pulses. Instead of returning to the starting position after each lunge, remain in the lunge position and perform small up and down pulses for a count of 10 before switching legs. This will engage your glutes and thighs even more intensely.

STEP 1

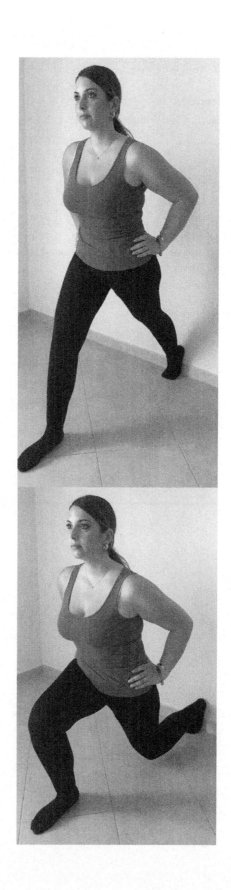

STEP 2

WALL-SUPPORTED PISTOL SQUATS

Total Time: 7 minutes

Equipment Needed:
- Exercise mat (optional)

Procedure:
1. Begin by standing with your back towards the wall and position yourself approximately 1 foot (30 cm) away from it.
2. Position your feet at a distance matching the width of your shoulders. This marks your initial stance.
3. Elevate your right leg, stretching it directly ahead. Keep your balance by grounding your left foot.
4. Slowly lower your body into a deep squat on your left leg, using the wall for support as needed. Your extended right leg should remain off the ground throughout the movement. Ensure you're engaging your glutes and legs throughout the movement.
5. Press through your left heel, activating your glutes and legs, to return to the starting position.
6. Repeat the movement with the opposite leg.

Repetitions and Rest:
- 4 sets x 5 reps (for each leg)
- Recovery: 60 seconds between sets

Advanced Variation: For an enhanced challenge, attempt the pistol squat without relying on the wall. Make sure to keep the focus on the glutes and legs throughout the exercise for maximum benefits.

STEP 1

STEP 2

STEP 3

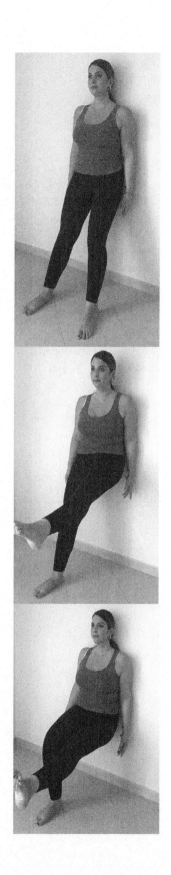

GLUTE BRIDGE WALL SLIDES

Total Time: 11 minutes

Equipment Needed:
- Exercise mat

Procedure:
1. Start by positioning yourself on your back on the workout mat, with your face turned towards the ceiling. Adjust your position so that your feet are pressed flat against the wall with your knees forming a 90-degree angle. Ensure you are around 2 feet (60 cm) away from the wall, allowing your feet to rest comfortably against it.
2. Place your arms at your sides, palms facing down for stability.
3. Press through your heels, lifting your hips off the ground and engaging your glutes. This is your bridge position.
4. While maintaining the bridge, slowly slide one foot upwards along the wall as high as your flexibility allows, keeping the other foot stationary. Ensure that you're engaging your glutes and hamstrings throughout this motion.
5. Slowly slide the raised foot back down to its starting position while maintaining the bridge.
6. Perform the action again using the other foot.

Repetitions and Rest:
- 3 sets x 10 reps (for each leg)
- Recovery: 45 seconds between sets

Advanced Variation: For added intensity, slide both feet up the wall simultaneously while maintaining the bridge position. This will demand extra engagement from the glutes and hamstrings and provide a more challenging core workout. Ensure proper form to prevent any strain.

STEP 1

STEP 2

STEP 3

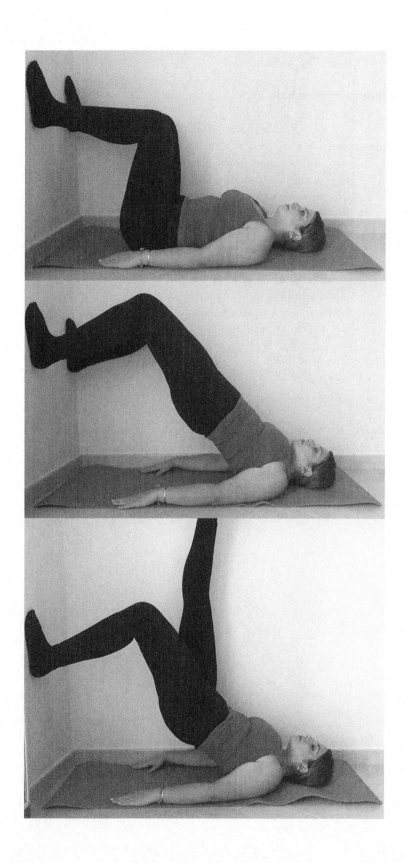

WALL SIDE LEG LIFTS

Total Time: 8 minutes

Equipment Needed:
- Exercise mat

Procedure:
1. Begin by aligning yourself laterally, around 1 foot (30cm) distant from the wall. Stand tall with the side of your right foot flat against the wall and your left foot firmly planted on the exercise mat.
2. Extend your right arm forward and place the palm against the wall for support, while extending your left arm out to the side for balance. Ensure your core is engaged.
3. Slowly lift your left leg up to the side as high as you comfortably can, ensuring you're engaging the muscles in the outer thigh and glutes. Make sure to keep your foot flexed and your toes pointing forward.
4. Gradually bring your leg down back to the initial position without allowing it to make contact with the floor. This motion will maximize the tension in the target muscles.
5. After completing the repetitions for one side, turn around so that the side of your left foot is against the wall. Extend your left arm forward with the palm against the wall, and extend your right arm out to the side. Perform the leg lift again using your right leg.

Repetitions and Rest:
- 3 sets x 12 reps (for each leg)
- Recovery: 30 seconds between sets

Advanced Variation: To intensify the workout, wear ankle weights while performing the leg lifts. This will add resistance, further challenging your glutes and thighs. Make sure to keep the correct posture and steer clear of any abrupt motions to avoid getting hurt.

STEP 1

STEP 2

WALL SQUAT WITH CALF RAISE

Total Time: 8 minutes

Equipment Needed:
- Exercise mat (optional)

Procedure:
1. Begin by positioning yourself parallel to a sturdy wall, about 2 feet (60 cm) away.
2. Position your feet so they are aligned with your shoulders Press your back evenly against the wall.
3. Slowly slide your back down the wall, lowering yourself into a squat position. Ensure that your thighs are aligned horizontally with the floor, with your knees positioned directly over your ankles. Maintain your back firmly against the wall throughout this exercise.
4. Upon achieving the squat posture, exert force through the front part of your feet, elevating your heels off the ground, which in turn engages your calf muscles. The body's weigh should be borne by the front part of your feet.
5. Gradually return your heels to the ground.
6. Press through your heels to slide back up the wall, returning to the standing position.

Repetitions and Rest:
- 3 sets x 15 reps
- Recovery: 40 seconds between sets

Advanced Variation: To increase the intensity, while in the squat position and after the calf raise, add a pulse. This means you'll lower your body a few inches more (deepening the squat) and then return to the parallel thigh position before sliding back up the wall. This extra movement intensifies the work on the glutes and thighs. Consistently ensure that your back is straight and the right form is upheld during the exercise.

STEP 1

STEP 2

STEP 3

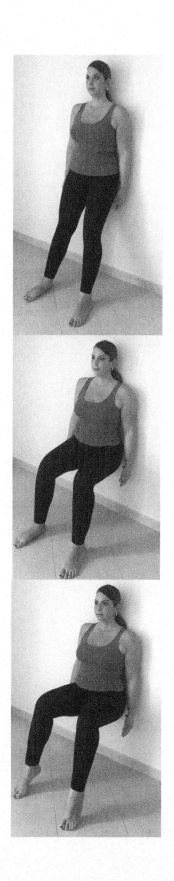

ELEVATED STALLION PULSES

Total Time: 8 minutes

Equipment Needed:
- Exercise mat

Procedure:
1. Begin by arranging your body so that your hands and knees make contact with the exercise mat. Ensure your knees are aligned directly under your hips, and your wrists are positioned beneath your shoulders. Curl your toes underneath you.
2. Shift your tailbone slightly forward to activate your core muscles. This positioning aids in supporting your lower back throughout the movement.
3. Carefully raise your knees from the mat, keeping them slightly elevated at just a few inches above. This alone can be a test of your stability and strength.
4. Once you've achieved a balanced and steady position, raise one foot towards the ceiling, keeping a firm 90-degree angle at the knee and pointing your toe elegantly.
5. Lower the leg until the knees are level, making sure not to let the foot touch the ground.
6. Pulse in this elevated position, raising and lowering your leg a few inches for enhanced muscle engagement.

Repetitions and Rest:
- 4 sets x 15 pulses (per side)
- Recovery: 20 seconds between sets

Advanced Variation: For an intensified burn, after completing the pulses on one side, hold the leg at its highest point and perform small circular rotations. This challenges both stability and muscle endurance, particularly targeting the glutes and hamstrings.

STEP 1

STEP 2

STEP 3

STEP 4

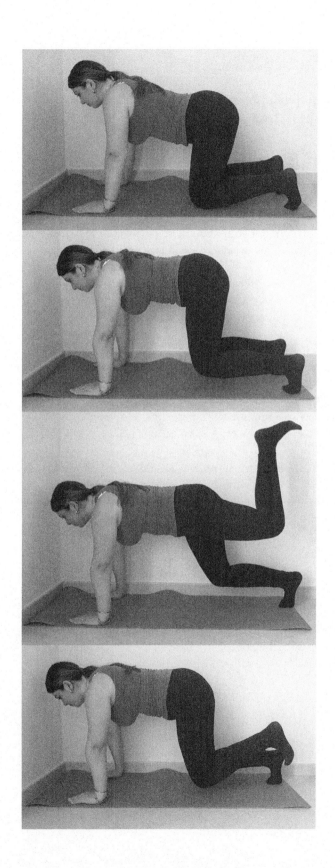

HIGH WALL GLUTE KICKBACKS

Total Time: 8 minutes

Equipment Needed:
- Exercise mat

Procedure:
1. Start by positioning the exercise mat perpendicular to a sturdy wall.
2. Instead of a traditional plank position, bend your knees, positioning them as if you're about to crawl. Your toes should be a few inches (or centimeters) away from the wall.
3. Place your forearms on the mat with hands closed in fists, ensuring they are shoulder-width apart and directly under your shoulders. This will be your base support.
4. Activate your core muscles while keeping your spine in a neutral position. Start moving your feet up the wall until your body and legs create an angle of 45 degrees (or more) with the ground. Ensure that only the front part of your feet makes contact with the wall.
5. Once stable, while keeping one foot pressed against the wall, raise the other leg, bending at the knee, and then kick straight back, targeting the glutes. Ensure your hips remain square to the mat and avoid any unnecessary rotation.
6. Slowly return the leg to its starting position against the wall.
7. Maintain the movement for the specified number of repetition before transitioning to the other leg

Repetitions and Rest:
- 3 sets x 12 kickbacks (per leg)
- Recovery: 15 seconds between sets.

Advanced Variation: For an added challenge, incorporate a resistance band around your thighs, just above the knees. This will provide additional resistance during the kickback motion and intensify the activation in the glutes. Ensure the band remains taut but not overly restrictive to facilitate a full range of motion.

STEP 1-2

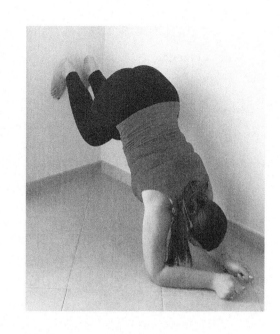

STEP 3-4

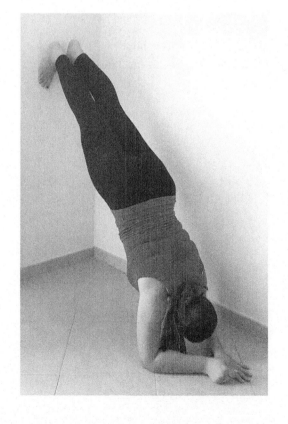

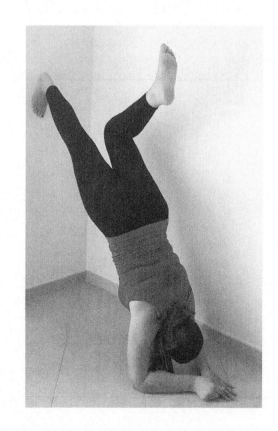

CHAPTER 7 - EXERCISES FOR ARMS AND SHOULDERS

WALL PUSH-UPS

Total Time: 7 minutes

Equipment Needed:
- None (a smooth wall surface is essential)

Procedure:
1. Stand upright facing a wall. Your feet should be approximately 2 feet (roughly 60 centimeters) away from the wall base.
2. Stretch out your arms in front of you and put your hands flat against the wall, positioning them a bit wider than the width of your shoulders. This will be your initial position.
3. Activate your central muscles, making sure your body maintains a straight alignment from your head to you heels.
4. Initiate the motion by flexing your elbows and inclining your body toward the wall. Ensure your elbows are angled slightly inward, not flaring outward.
5. Keep moving forward until your nose is nearly in contact with the wall.
6. Breathe out and return to the initial position by extending your arms. Ensure your body remains aligned and your core is active during the whole action.

Repetitions and Rest:
- 3 sets x 15 reps
- Recovery: 45 seconds between sets

Advanced Variation: To increase the intensity of the Wall Push-up, position your feet further away from the wall. This alteration increases the angle and demands more strength from the arms and shoulders. Another variant is to elevate one leg off the ground while performing the push-up, challenging the core and balance even more.

STEP 1

STEP 2

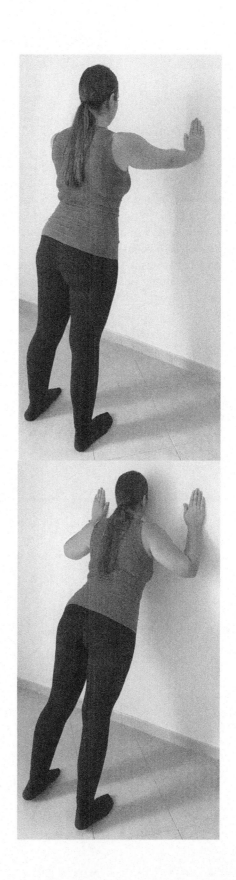

ISOMETRIC WALL PRESS

Total Time: 5 minutes

Equipment Needed:
- A sturdy wall

Procedure:
1. Stand upright and face the wall. The distance should be close enough to where you can extend your arms fully and place your palms flat on the wall without leaning forward.
2. Put your hands on the wall, level with your chest, and set them a bit beyond shoulder width. Spread your fingers wide, ensuring the entire palm and fingers maintain firm contact with the wall.
3. Activate your central muscles and maintain a straight spine. Make sure your feet are spaced the width of your hips and are solidly on the ground.
4. Press into the wall as if you're trying to push it away from you, but without actually moving. This is an isometric contraction, meaning the muscle length doesn't change and there's no visible movement in the arms.
5. Hold this press while maintaining a tight core and controlled breathing. Keep your neck neutral and your gaze forward.

Repetitions and Rest:
- 4 sets x 20 seconds press
- Recovery: 30 seconds between sets

Advanced Variation: To ramp up the challenge, perform the Isometric Wall Press on a single arm. Position yourself slightly to the side of the wall so that you can press with one hand while the other hand remains at your side or on your hip. This not only intensifies the arm and shoulder workout but also demands more from your core to maintain balance and posture.

SINGLE STEP

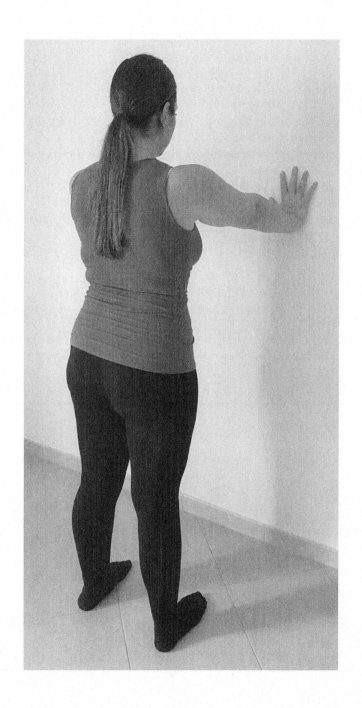

DIAMOND WALL PUSH-UPS

Total Time: 7 minutes

Equipment Needed:
- A sturdy wall
- Exercise mat (optional for added grip)

Procedure:
1. Stand upright facing the wall. Begin at a distance from the wall the lets you stretch out your arms completely, with your palms laying flat on the wall.
2. Move your hands towards each other on the wall, creating a diamond shape by touching your thumbs and index fingers together. Your hands should be at chest height.
3. Position your feet hip-width apart with your heels grounded. Activate your central muscles and maintain a straight alignment of your spine.
4. Breathe in while your flex your elbows, drawing your torso nearer to the wall. Make sure your elbows angle outwards as you descend smoothly.
5. Breathe out as you push away, straightening your arms to go back to the initial stance.

Repetitions and Rest:
- 4 sets x 12 reps
- Recovery: 40 seconds between sets

Advanced Variation: To further challenge yourself, shift your feet further back from the wall, increasing the angle of your body. This adjustment increases the bodyweight resistance and targets the muscles with more intensity. Ensure that as you move back, the diamond hand placement remains consistent and your form is not compromised.

STEP 1

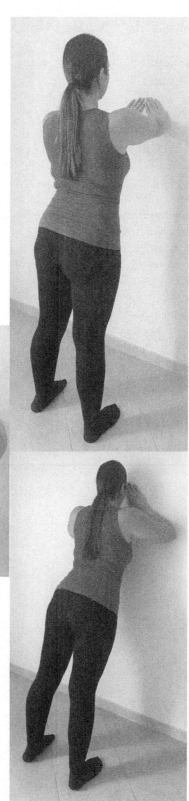

HAND POSITIONING

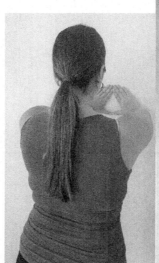

STEP 2

WALL-SUPPORTED PLANK TO PIKE

Total Time: 9 minutes

Equipment Needed:
- A sturdy wall
- Exercise mat

Procedure:
1. Begin by placing the exercise mat perpendicular to the wall. Begin by getting into a plank posture with your feet joined together, and toes placed close to the bottom of the wall.
2. Stretch your arms out completely, with your hands placed right under your shoulders on the mat. Ensure a straight-line posture from your head to your heels.
3. Engage your core muscles to maintain a stable hip position, neither sagging nor lifted too high. Keep your gaze downward towards the floor.
4. As you inhale, use your core muscles and legs to push your feet up the wall, simultaneously lifting your hips toward the ceiling and forming an inverted "V" or pike position with your body. Your hands remain stationary on the mat.
5. At the peak of the movement, your body will resemble an upside-down "V", with your heels gently resting on the wall and the balls of your feet supporting most of the weight.
6. Exhale as you gradually lower your body back to the plank position, controlling the descent with your core.

Repetitions and Rest:
- 4 sets x 10 reps
- Recovery: 45 seconds between sets

Advanced Variation: For those looking for a greater challenge, after returning to the plank position, perform a push-up. This not only intensifies the core work during the pike but also incorporates strength training for the arms and chest. Ensure you maintain proper form throughout to prevent strain or injury.

STEP 1

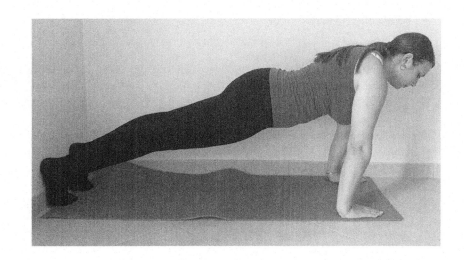

STEP 2

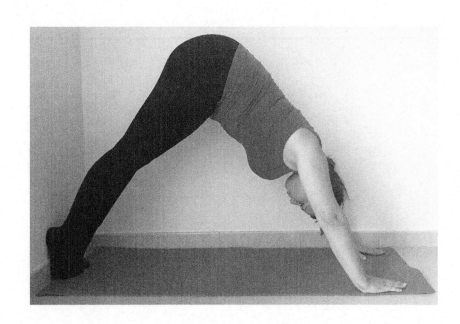

WALL LATERAL RAISE SLIDES

Total Time: 8 minutes

Equipment Needed:
- Exercise mat (optional)
- Smooth wall surface

Procedure:
1. Stand upright and position yourself with your right side facing the wall, with your feet placed about 12 inches (30 cm) away from the baseboard.
2. Extend your right arm straight out to your side, ensuring your palm is facing the wall and your fingertips are touching it.
3. Ensure your feet are securely positioned on the ground and engage your core muscles. This will serve as your initial stance.
4. Begin the movement by sliding your hand up the wall, raising your arm as high as you can. As you do this, allow your arm to move slightly backward in relation to the rest of your body, but ensure you're not arching your back.
5. Slowly slide your hand back down to the starting position, controlling the descent. This completes one repetition.
6. After completing the designated number of reps on one side, switch to face the opposite direction, and repeat with your left arm.

Repetitions and Rest:
- 3 sets x 12 reps
- Recovery: 30 seconds between sets

Advanced Variation: To increase the intensity and further challenge the shoulder muscles, loop a light resistance band around your wrist and secure the other end under your foot on the same side. As your lift your arm, the resistance band will offer extra tension. This will require more strength and stability during the lateral raise movement. Ensure the resistance band is suitable for your strength level to avoid overexertion or strain.

STEP 1

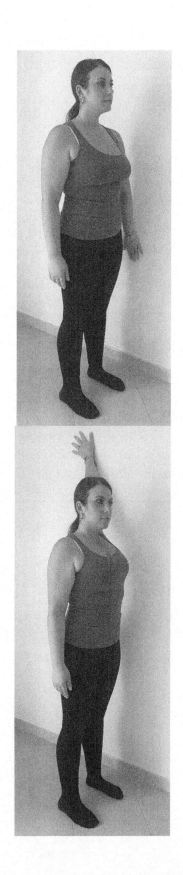

STEP 2

WALL PLANK ARM CIRCLES

Total Time: 8 minutes

Equipment Needed:
- None

Procedure:
1. Start by standing about 2 feet (60 cm) away from the wall.
2. Position yourself facing the wall, lean forward, and set your hands against it at shoulder level, spaced shoulder-width apart, transitioning into a modified plank stance. Your body should exhibit a straight alignment from head to heels.
3. Press through the palms to engage the shoulders and core.
4. Lift your right hand off the wall and start making small circles in the air – first clockwise for the count of 8 and then counter-clockwise for the count of 8.
5. Place the right hand back on the wall and repeat with the left hand.
6. Ensure your core is tight and hips are squared throughout the exercise. Try to keep the rest of your body stationary and avoid any excessive movement in the hips.

Repetitions and Rest:
- 3 sets x 8 reps (One rep includes circles in both directions for one arm)
- Recovery: 30 seconds between sets

Advanced Variation: To make this exercise more challenging, you can:
- Stand on one leg while performing the arm circles, switching legs with each set.
- Increase the size of the circles or the duration (e.g., making circles for a count of 16 or 20).
- Combine it with a wall push-up between each arm circle set.

This exercise will help in strengthening the arms, shoulders, and core muscles while also improving stability and balance.

STEP 1

STEP 2

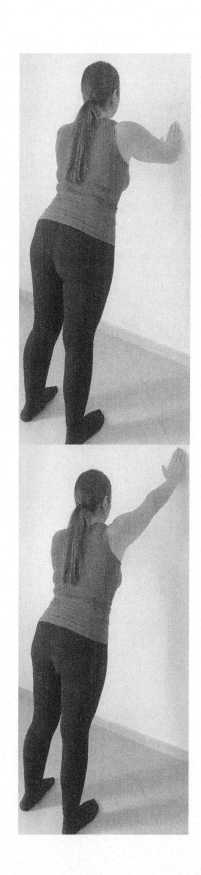

WALL WALKS

Total Time: 6 minutes

Equipment Needed:
- None

Procedure:
1. Begin by standing with your back to the wall, a few feet away (about 2 feet or 60 cm). Position your feet shoulder-width apart.
2. Lean forward from your hips, placing your palms flat on the floor with a distance about as wide as your shoulders between them.
3. Gradually start moving your feet up the wall while at the same time moving your hands closer to the wall. Your goal is to get as vertical as possible, ideally aiming for a handstand position or as close to it as your strength and flexibility allow.
4. Once you've reached your highest point, start the descent: walk your hands away from the wall while walking your feet down the wall until you return to the starting position. That completes one rep.

Repetitions and Rest:
- 3 sets x 3 reps
- Recovery: 45 seconds between sets

Advanced Variation: Once you've walked into the vertical position, try holding for a few seconds (3-5 seconds) before starting your descent. This adds an isometric component to the exercise, further challenging the shoulders and core.

STEP 1

STEP 2

WALL-SUPPORTED SIDE PLANK WITH ARM RAISE

Total Time: 8 minutes

Equipment Needed:
- None

Procedure:
1. Begin by positioning yourself on your right side with extended legs, and place your feet against the wall's base.
2. Lift yourself up on your right elbow, making sure it's aligned directly beneath your shoulder. Your body should exhibit a straight alignment from head to heels.
3. Press the palm of your feet against the wall for added stability.
4. Extend your right arm, placing your right hand flat on the ground for extra balance.
5. Lift your left arm upward slowly until it's at a right angle to the ground. As you do this, keep your eyes following your left hand, ensuring your chest, torso, and hips remain square and do not sag or rotate.
6. Hold this side plank with arm raise position for the required time.
7. Lower the left arm back down and switch sides to repeat the procedure on the left side.

Repetitions and Rest:
- 4 sets x 15 seconds per side
- Recovery: 30 seconds between sets

Advanced Variation: As your left arm is raised, simultaneously lift your left leg a few inches off the right leg, holding it in the air for the duration of the plank.

STEP 1

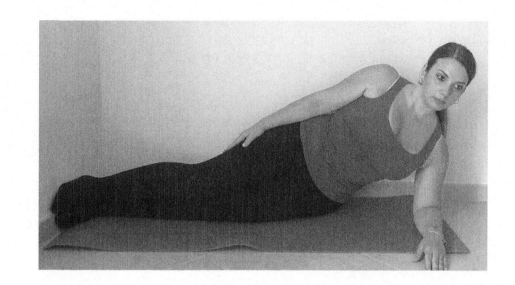

STEP 2

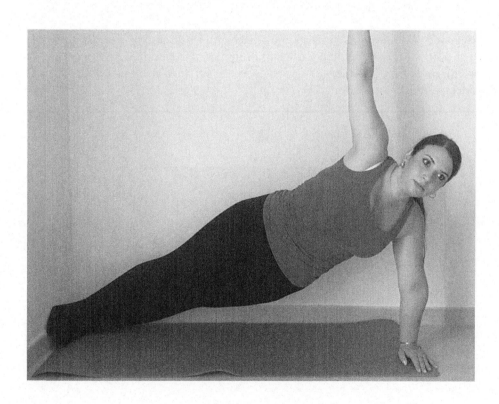

CHAPTER 8 - EXERCISES FOR FLEXIBILITY AND BALANCE

WALL-ASSISTED DEEP LUNGE STRETCH

Total Time: 7 minutes

Equipment Needed:
- Exercise mat (optional but recommended for comfort)

Procedure:
1. Stand with your back to the wall, ensuring there's enough space in front of you to lunge forward.
2. Step forward with your right foot, approximately 3 feet (about 90 cm) away from the wall.
3. Bend the right knee to a 90-degree angle, ensuring your right knee is aligned over your right ankle.
4. The left foot should slide back, toes pointing downward, with the ball of the foot and the toes pressing into the wall. Your left leg should be extended straight.
5. Drop your hips down and forward to deepen the stretch, feeling it in the front of your left hip and thigh.
6. Keep the upper body straight with your hands on your hips or raised overhead for an added stretch.
7. Maintain this position and breathe deeply, ensuring the hips remain square and facing forward.

Repetitions and Rest:
- 4 sets x 30 seconds per leg
- Recovery: 15 seconds between sets

Advanced Variation: To intensify the stretch, after positioning yourself in the deep lunge, place your opposite hand (if the right foot is forward, use the left hand) on the ground beside your front foot. Twist your torso and raise the other arm (right arm, in this case) towards the ceiling, looking up at your raised hand. This not only deepens the hip stretch but also introduces a spinal rotation for added flexibility.

STEP 1

STEP 2

WALL BRIDGE EXTENSIONS

Total Time: 8 minutes

Equipment Needed:
- Exercise mat

Procedure:
1. Begin by lying flat on your back on the exercise mat, positioning yourself so that your feet are flat against the wall. The distance should be such that your legs form a 90-degree angle at the knees, roughly 1.5 to 2 feet (45 to 60 cm) away from the wall.
2. Extend your arms alongside your body, palms facing down.
3. Activate your abdominal muscles and push your feet against the wall as you raise your hips from the floor. As you do this, ensure that you're pressing through the shoulders and arms to get maximum elevation.
4. Once your body forms a straight line from your shoulders to the knees, extend one leg straight out while keeping the other foot pressing into the wall.
5. Hold the leg extension for a moment, then return the foot to the wall.
6. Return your hips to the starting position by lowering them back down.
7. Repeat the bridge lift and leg extension using the opposite leg.

Repetitions and Rest:
- 3 sets x 10 reps (5 reps per leg)
- Recovery: 20 seconds between sets

Advanced Variation: After you've raised your hips and are in the bridge position with one leg extended, introduce a small circular motion with the extended leg, making 5 circles clockwise and 5 counterclockwise before returning the foot to the wall and lowering the hips. This not only challenges your hip muscles but also enhances your balance and core stability.

STEP 1

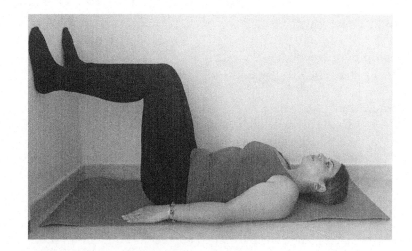

STEP 2

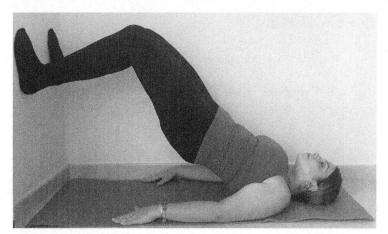

STEP 3

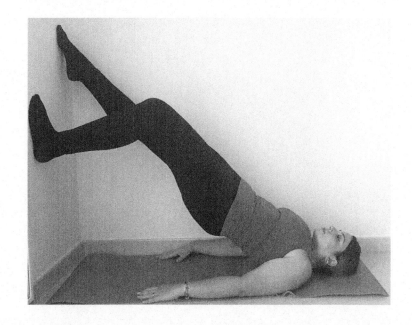

WALL-SUPPORTED SINGLE LEG SQUATS

Total Time: 6 minutes

Equipment Needed:
- Exercise mat (optional for added comfort)

Procedure:
1. Stand with your back to the wall, at a distance of approximately 2 feet (60 cm).
2. Lean back slightly until your upper back makes gentle contact with the wall.
3. Place your feet hip-width apart, ensuring they are flat on the ground.
4. Raise your right knee toward your chest, ensuring your left foot remains solidly planted on the floor.
5. Slowly bend your left knee, performing a single leg squat.
6. Engage your core muscles and keep your spine erect. Your left leg should bear most of your weight.
7. Maintaining control, bring your right leg back down to its starting position.
8. After completing the desired number of leg lifts with your right leg, switch to your left leg and repeat the motion.

Repetitions and Rest:
- 3 sets x 12 reps (per leg)
- Recovery: 20 seconds between sets

Advanced Variation: In order to intensify the challenge, clutch a light dumbbell or kettlebell near your chest while executing the squat. Make certain the weight is handleable, and your posture stays correct throughout the workout.

STEP 1

STEP 2

STEP 3

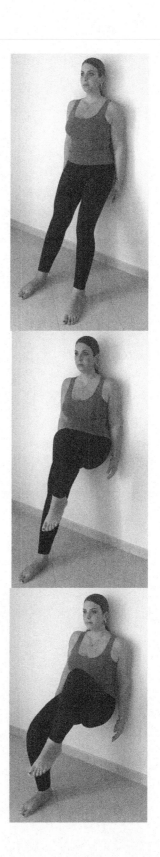

STANDING WALL SINGLE-LEG BALANCE

Total Time: 6 minutes

Equipment Needed:
- Exercise mat (optional for added comfort)

Procedure:
1. Stand with your back to the wall, positioning yourself approximately 1 foot (30 cm) away.
2. Plant one foot firmly on the ground and find a stable and comfortable stance. This will be your supporting leg.
3. Slowly lift the other leg off the ground, bending at the knee to form a 90-degree angle. Your lifted foot can rest against the opposite knee, forming a figure-four position.
4. Extend your arms outward to the sides for balance. If you're having trouble maintaining balance, you can lightly press your hands against the wall for additional support.
5. Engage your core muscles and focus on maintaining a straight posture. Avoid tilting to one side or allowing your hips to droop.
6. Hold this single-leg stance while maintaining your balance and posture. Breathe steadily and avoid locking the knee of the supporting leg.
7. After the desired hold time, switch legs and repeat the process.

Repetitions and Rest:
- 3 sets x 30 seconds per leg
- Recovery: 15 seconds between sets

Advanced Variation: To challenge your balance further, close your eyes while holding the single-leg stance. This eliminates visual cues and forces your body to rely more on proprioception (sense of body position) for balance. Make sure you're near the wall so that you can lean on it for assistance if necessary.

STEP 1

STEP 2

WALL-SUPPORTED WARRIOR III STRETCH

Total Time: 7 minutes

Equipment Needed:
- Exercise mat (optional for added comfort)

Procedure:
1. Start by standing upright approximately 3-4 feet (90-120 centimeters) away from a solid wall.
2. Lean forward, positioning your hands on the wall at a level equal to your shoulders and spaced apart at the width of your shoulders. Be certain that there is a 90-degree angle between your back and legs.
3. Shift your weight onto your right foot, ensuring it is firmly grounded and centered.
4. Slowly lift your left leg behind you while keeping it straight. Try to elevate it to the level of your hip or as far as your flexibility permits. Your body should create a "T" shape, with the foot on the ground serving as the foundation.
5. While raising the leg, activate your core muscles to uphold stability and maintain the pelvis in a neutral position, preventing it from tilting to the side. Your toes should point downward, and the foot remains flexed.
6. Extend your chest forward while keeping your spine long, gazing downward and slightly ahead.
7. Hold the position, maintaining a strong, engaged core, and ensuring even breathing.

Repetitions and Rest:
- 4 sets x 30 seconds per leg
- Recovery: 15 seconds between sets

Advanced Variation: To increase the challenge:
- Once comfortable with the basic Wall-Supported Warrior III Stretch, try lifting the hands off the wall and extending them forward, parallel to the ground, while balancing on one foot.
- Engage the core and back muscles to maintain the "T" shape, ensuring that the raised leg, torso, and arms remain parallel to the ground.
- Hold this position without wall support for the desired time, and then switch legs. Remember always to keep the core engaged and the spine long for balance and support.

STEP 1

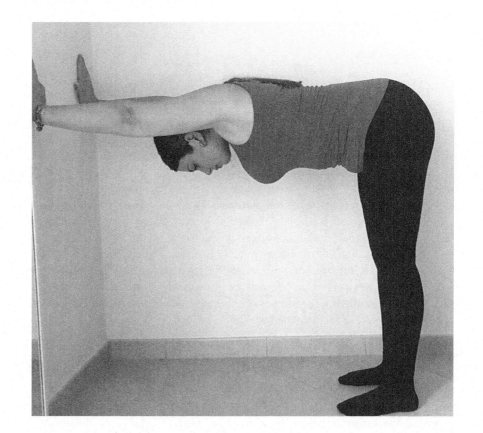

STEP 2

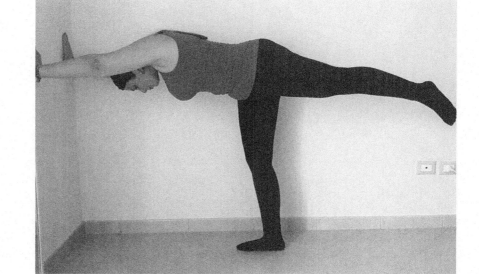

WALL-SUPPORTED TREE POSE STRETCH

Total Time: 5 minutes

Equipment Needed:
- Exercise mat

Procedure:
1. Start by positioning yourself sideways approximately 2 feet (60 centimeters) away from the wall. The wall should be nearer to your right side.
2. Ground your left foot solidly onto the floor. Your feet should be positioned with a gap equal to the width of your hips to establish a solid foundation.
3. Transfer most of your body weight onto your left foot.
4. Softly curve your right knee and raise the underside of your right foot. Position it against either the inner left calf or the inner left thigh. Avoid placing the foot against your knee to prevent undue stress.
5. Once you've achieved a comfortable foot placement, use the wall as a support by resting your right hand or elbow on it. This will assist with balance.
6. Keep your left hand on your waist or raise it towards the sky, fingers pointing upwards.
7. Make sure your back is aligned, and fix your eyes on a stable point ahead of you to aid in keeping your balance.
8. After completing the stretch on one side, switch to the other side by positioning your left side closer to the wall and repeating the process with the left leg.

Repetitions and Rest:
- 3 sets x 30 seconds per side
- Recovery: 15 seconds between sets

Advanced Variation: For those looking for an added challenge:
- Try performing the pose without using the wall for support. Begin with a hand on the wall, then gradually attempt to lift your hand off, only using it when needed for stability.
- As you progress, lift both hands to meet overhead in a prayer position, deepening the stretch and testing your balance further.

STEP 1

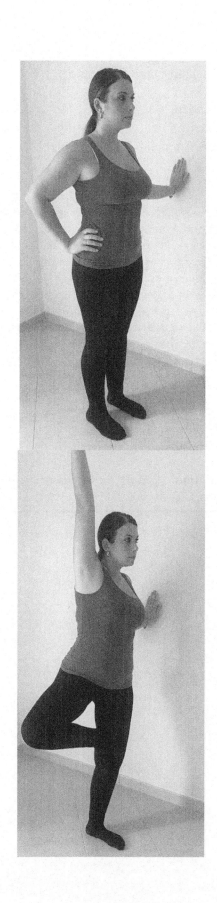

STEP 2

T-SPINE WALL STRETCH

Total Time: 5 minutes

Equipment Needed:
- Wall space
- Exercise mat (optional for comfort)

Procedure:
1. Stand facing the wall, roughly 1 foot (30 centimeters) away.
2. Spread your feet shoulder-width apart for a stable stance.
3. Stretch both your arms forward so they are level with the ground.
4. Place your palms flat against the wall, keeping them shoulder-width apart.
5. Start moving your hands up the wall until they're completely stretched out over your head. Your hands should remain flat against the wall throughout this motion.
6. As you extend upward, pivot at the hips and incline towards the wall. Your head should move between your arms, allowing a deep stretch in the thoracic spine region.
7. Maintain a neutral neck by looking downward, ensuring your cervical spine is in line with the rest of your back.
8. Push gently into the wall with your hands while sinking your chest toward the floor, accentuating the stretch in the upper back.
9. Breathe deeply and evenly, letting any tension in your mid-back region release.

Repetitions and Rest:
- 4 sets x 40 seconds stretch
- Recovery: 20 seconds between sets

Advanced Variation: As you're in the stretch position with your arms extended and your head between your arms, try gently rotating your torso to one side and then the other. This will give a rotational stretch to the thoracic spine, adding a dynamic component to the stretch. Ensure that the movement is controlled, and avoid over-rotating. Always return to the center before rotating to the opposite side.

STEP 1

STEP 2

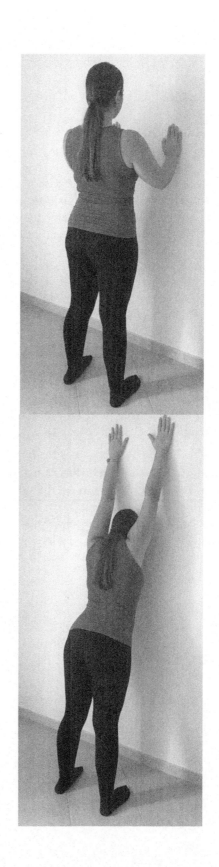

WALL SPLIT PROGRESSIONS

Total Time: 8 minutes

Equipment Needed:
- Wall space
- Exercise mat

Procedure:
1. Begin by lying down on the mat with your back flat on the floor and your buttocks positioned close to the wall.
2. Adjust your position so that your glutes are almost touching the wall.
3. Extend both legs up and rest them straight against the wall, forming an "L" shape with your body.
4. Spread your legs out to the sides, going as wide as your flexibility allows. This is your starting position for the wall split.
5. Press the backs of your thighs and calves against the wall as you let gravity assist in pushing your legs further apart. You should feel a stretch in the inner thighs.
6. Hold the stretch, taking deep breaths and allowing the legs to naturally fall wider with each exhale.
7. After holding for the desired time, use your hands to assist in bringing the legs back to the center and then lower them down.

Repetitions and Rest:
- 3 sets x 15 reps
- Recovery: 20 seconds between sets

Advanced Variation: To intensify the stretch and challenge your flexibility further:
- From the starting position, flex your feet, actively pressing the heels into the wall.
- Activate your core muscles while maintaining your back pressed against the mat.
- As you spread your legs apart for the split, instead of letting gravity do all the work, actively push your legs wider using your leg muscles.

This active engagement will not only stretch the inner thighs more intensely but also strengthen the surrounding muscles. Remember to maintain a steady breathing pattern and not to push beyond your limits.

STEP 1

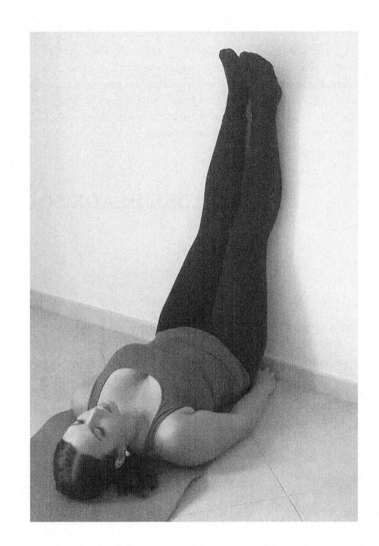

STEP 2

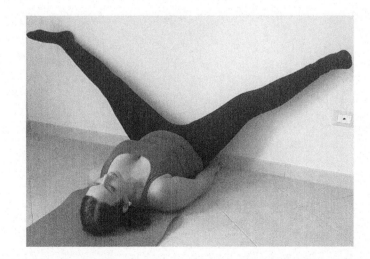

CHAPTER 9 - EXERCISES FOR PERFECT POSTURE

While the exercises described in previous chapters, including the stretches and those targeting the core muscles, undeniably play a pivotal role in enhancing one's posture, they are just part of the posture-improving puzzle. Flexibility exercises, along with core-strengthening routines, are instrumental in maintaining spinal alignment and promoting an upright stance. However, to truly unlock impeccable posture, there are four indispensable exercises that zero in on the muscles of the upper body, particularly focusing on the back, trapezius, and shoulder muscles. These exercises aren't merely an adjunct to your routine; they are fundamental. In this chapter, we'll delve deep into these four transformative exercises, granting you the key to perfect posture.

SHOULDER BLADE SQUEEZE

Total Time: 5 minutes

Equipment Needed:
- Wall space

Procedure:
1. Maintain an upright posture with your back pressed straight against the wall. Your feet should be about shoulder-width apart and approximately 6 inches (15 centimeters) away from the wall.
2. Reach your arms straight ahead at shoulder height, palms facing each other.
3. Begin the movement by opening your arms out to the sides, aiming to bring your shoulder blades as close together as possible without causing discomfort. As you do this, rotate your arms so the back of your hands approach and eventually make contact with the wall.
4. Hold this position for a few seconds, feeling the muscles between your shoulder blades engaging.
5. Slowly return your arms to the starting position in front of you, maintaining a controlled motion throughout.

Repetitions and Rest:
- 3 sets x 15 reps
- Recovery: 20 seconds between sets

Advanced Variation: For those looking to elevate the intensity of the Shoulder Blade Squeeze, try adding a resistance band. Starting with both hands holding the band in front of you, pull the band apart as you squeeze your shoulder blades together and open your arms out to the sides. This adds resistance, further engaging the muscles and amplifying the benefits. Ensure the movement is controlled, and the focus remains on the shoulder blade squeeze.

STEP 1

STEP 2

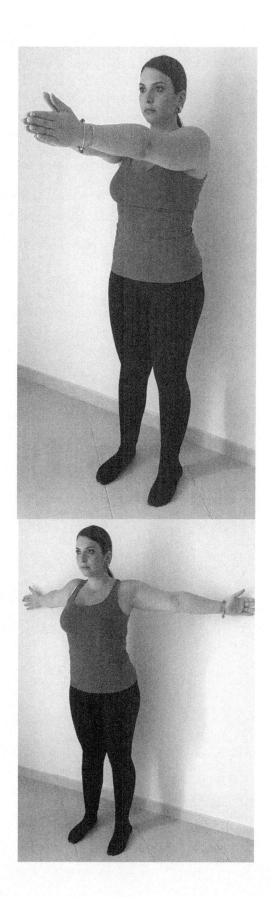

WALL ANGELS

Total Time: 5 minutes

Equipment Needed:
- Wall space

Procedure:
1. Ensure your back is flat against the wall. Your feet should be shoulder-width apart and positioned approximately 2 inches (5 centimeters) away from the wall.
2. Bend your knees slightly to ensure a neutral spine position.
3. Press the back of your head, upper back, and tailbone into the wall. The designated points should remain in touch with the wall during the entire exercise.
4. Position your arms in a "W" shape with the back of your hands, forearms, and elbows pressed firmly against the wall.
5. In a controlled motion, slide your arms upward into an "I" shape, maintaining contact between the back of your arms and the wall. If you're unable to keep contact at first, go as far as your mobility allows.
6. Once you reach the top of the motion, slowly slide your arms back down to the initial "W" position.

Repetitions and Rest:
- 3 sets x 10 reps
- Recovery: 20 seconds between sets

Advanced Variation: For a heightened challenge, incorporate a resistance band looped around both wrists. As you move your arms from the "I" to the "W" position, the band will add resistance, requiring additional strength and stability to maintain the movement. Ensure that the resistance level of the band complements your strength and does not compromise form.

STEP 1

STEP 2

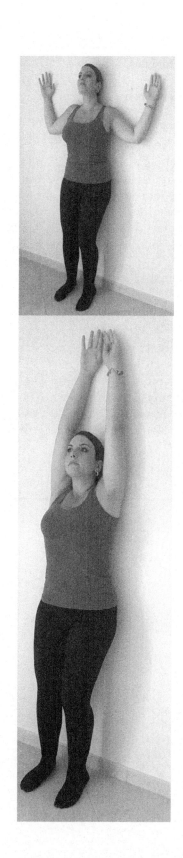

CHIN TUCKS AGAINST THE WALL

Total Time: 4 minutes

Equipment Needed:
Wall space

Procedure:
1. Stand upright with your back and heels flush against the wall. Your feet should be shoulder-width apart.
2. Confirm that your shoulders are at ease and your arms are hanging freely by your sides.
3. Stretch out your spine and push the back part of your head against the wall. Your body should exhibit a straight alignment from head to tailbone.
4. Softly draw your chin towards your chest, aiming to create a double chin. While doing this, press the back of your neck against the wall, but ensure you don't strain or force it. This action activates the muscles at the front of your neck.
5. Maintain the tucked chin position for a brief duration, then relax and revert to the initial position.

Repetitions and Rest:
- 3 sets x 10 reps
- Recovery: 15 seconds between sets

Advanced Variation: For those seeking an enhanced challenge, try the seated chin tucks against the wall. Position yourself on the floor with your legs stretched out before you. Recline backwards until both your upper back and the back of your head make contact with the wall. Ensure your lower back is not arched. Perform the chin tucks from this seated position. This alteration enhances the range of movement and engages more stabilizing muscle.

STEP 1

STEP 2

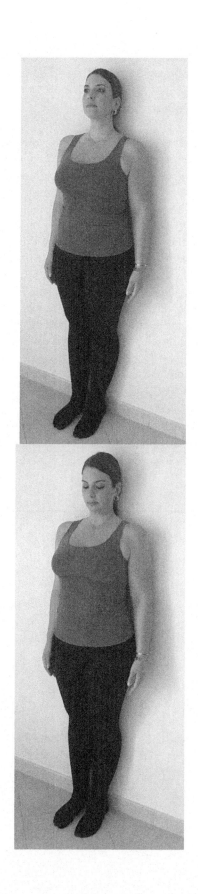

SIDE WALL ARM STRETCH

Total Time: 7 minutes

Equipment Needed:
- Wall space

Procedure:
1. Stand sideways to the wall, positioning your right side closer to it. Position your feet at a distance equal to the width of your shoulders, and about 6 inches (15 centimeters) away from the wall.
2. Extend your arms forward at shoulder level, with your palms facing one another.
3. Keeping your arms at shoulder height, slowly rotate your upper body to the left. As you do this, move your left arm outward towards the wall until the back of your left hand makes contact with it. Ensure that the movement is controlled and that you maintain the alignment of your spine throughout.
4. Once the back of your left hand touches the wall, hold the position for a few seconds, feeling the stretch along the left side of your torso and arm.
5. Gently revert to the initial stance with your palms in contact.
6. Repeat the same motion for the other side by switching your position so that your left side is now closer to the wall and moving your right arm towards it.

Repetitions and Rest:
- 3 sets x 10 reps per side
- Recovery: 15 seconds between sets

Advanced Variation: To add an extra challenge and further stretch the muscles, try holding each side stretch for a longer duration, such as 15-20 seconds. This will not only enhance flexibility but also improve endurance in the stretched muscles.

STEP 1

STEP 2

CHAPTER 10: 28-DAY CHALLENGE TO TRANSFORM YOUR BODY

In the fitness realm, there's a prevalent misbelieve that transformation necessitates a rapid, drastic shift. The truth is, consistent and dedicated effort over time is the magic formula. From the day you lace up your shoes and start your journey with Wall Pilates, every drop of sweat, every stretch, and every moment of mindfulness counts towards your transformation. Every day of the program has been meticulously crafted to provide a comprehensive routine with balanced exercises. As the days roll by, you'll notice the program ratcheting up in intensity. On certain days, we suggest undertaking the exercises in their advanced variations to really amp up the results. Nonetheless, it's vital to understand that each person commences from a unique position. If the advanced version feels too intense or doesn't match your current fitness level, please feel free to revert to the classic version. There's no shame in pacing yourself.

You're not just setting yourself up for a 28-day challenge; you're laying the foundation for lifelong fitness habits. This 28-day journey is a stepping stone towards the continuous transformation that your body will undergo month after month. But let's get one thing straight – while looking in the mirror and appreciating the toned glutes or the sculpted abs is a thrilling experience, this program goes beyond the surface. It delves deep into your well-being, amplifying your strength, flexibility, and endurance. It's not just about how you look; it's about how you feel, how you move, and how you tackle everyday challenges with newfound energy and confidence.

The 28-Days Blueprint

	CORE	LEGS & GLUTES	ARMS & SHOULDERS	FLEXIBILITY & BALANCE	POSTURE
Day 1	Core-Engaging Wall Squat – p. 24	Wall-Assisted Leg Circles – p. 28	Isometric Wall Press – p. 68	Wall Bridge Extensions – p. 84	Shoulder Blade Squeeze – p. 98
Day 2	Wall-Powered Plank Reach – p. 18	Standing Wall Leg Lifts – p. 22	Diamond Wall Push-Ups – p. 70	Wall-Assisted Deep Lunge Stretch – p. 82	Wall Angels – p. 100
Day 3	Wall Slide Shoulder Elevations – p. 26	Glute Bridge Wall Press – p. 20	Wall Plank Arm Circles – p. 76	Wall-Supported Tree Pose Stretch – p. 92	Chin Tucks Against The Wall – p. 102
Day 4	Standing Wall Twist – p. 30	Single-Leg Wall Push-Off – p. 32	Wall Walks – p. 78	Wall-Supported Warrior III Stretch – p. 90	Side Wall Arm Stretch – p. 104
Day 5	Isometric Wall Plank Hold – p. 36	Wall Squat With Calf Raise – p. 60	Wall Push-Ups – p. 66	Wall-Supported Single Leg Squats – p. 86	Shoulder Blade Squeeze – p. 98
Day 6	Wall Dead Bug – p. 44	Elevated Stallion Pulses – p. 62	Wall-Supported Plank To Pike – p. 72	Standing Wall Single-Leg Balance – p. 88	Wall Angels – p. 100
Day 7	Wall Mountain Climbers – p. 34	Elevated Wall Lunges – p. 52	Wall Lateral Raise Slides – p. 74	Wall Split Progressions – p. 96	Chin Tucks Against The Wall – p. 102
Day 8	Wall Leg Raises – p. 38	Glute Bridge Wall Slides – p. 56	Wall-Supported Side Plank With Arm Raise – p. 80	T-Spine Wall Stretch – p. 94	Side Wall Arm Stretch – p. 104
Day 9	Wall Dead Bug With Arm Slide – p. 46	Wall Side Leg Lifts – p. 58	Wall Walk (Advanced Variation) – p. 78	Wall-Supported Tree Pose Stretch (Advanced Variation) – p. 92	Shoulder Blade Squeeze – p. 98
Day 10	Wall Oblique Crunches – p. 40	Wall-Supported Pistol Squats – p. 54	Wall Push-Ups (Advanced Variation) – p. 66	Wall Bridge Extensions – p. 84	Wall Angels (Advanced Variation) – p. 100

Day 11	Vertical Wall Sit & Twist – p. 42	Wall Squat Holds – p. 50	Wall-Supported Side Plank With Arm Raise – p. 80	Wall-Assisted Deep Lunge Stretch (Advanced Variation) – p. 82	Chin Tucks Against The Wall – p. 102
Day 12	High Wall Knee Tucks – p. 48	High Wall Glute Kickbacks – p. 64	Wall Lateral Raise Slides (Advanced Variation) – p. 74	Standing Wall Single-Leg Balance (Advanced Variation) – p. 88	Side Wall Arm Stretch – p. 104
Day 13	Isometric Wall Plank Hold (Advanced Variation) – p. 36	Wall Squat With Calf Raise (Advanced Variation) – p. 60	Isometric Wall Press – p. 68	Wall-Supported Warrior III Stretch – p. 90	Shoulder Blade Squeeze (Advanced Variation) – p. 98
Day 14	Wall Dead Bug (Advanced Variation) – p. 44	Glute Bridge Wall Slides – p.56	Diamond Wall Push-Ups (Advanced Variation) – p. 70	T-Spine Wall Stretch – p. 94	Wall Angels – p. 100
Day 15	Wall Leg Raises – p. 38	Elevated Wall Lunges – p. 52	Wall Plank Arm Circles – p. 76	Wall-Supported Single Leg Squats (Advanced Variation) – p. 86	Chin Tucks Against The Wall (Advanced Variation) – p. 102
Day 16	Wall Mountain Climbers (Advanced Variation) – p. 34	High Wall Glute Kickbacks (Advanced Variation) – p. 64	Wall-Supported Plank To Pike (Advanced Variation) – p. 72	Wall Split Progressions – p. 96	Side Wall Arm Stretch – p. 104
Day 17	Wall Dead Bug With Arm Slide – p. 46	Wall Squat Holds (Advanced Variation) – p. 50	Isometric Wall Press (Advanced Variation) – p. 68	Wall Bridge Extensions (Advanced Variation) – p. 84	Shoulder Blade Squeeze – p. 98
Day 18	Vertical Wall Sit & Twist (Advanced Variation) – p. 42	Wall-Supported Pistol Squats – p. 54	Wall Walks (Advanced Variation) – p. 78	Standing Wall Single-Leg Balance – p. 88	Wall Angels (Advanced Variation) – p. 100
Day 19	High Wall Knee Tucks – p. 48	Wall Side Leg Lifts (Advanced Variation) – p. 58	Wall-Supported Side Plank With Arm Raise (Advanced Variation) – p. 80	Wall-Supported Warrior III Stretch (Advanced Variation) – p. 90	Chin Tucks Against The Wall (Advanced Variation) – p. 102
Day 20	Wall Oblique Crunches (Advanced Variation) – p. 40	Elevated Stallion Pulses (Advanced Variation) – p. 62	Wall Lateral Raise Slides – p. 74	T-Spine Wall Stretch (Advanced Variation) – p. 94	Side Wall Arm Stretch (Advanced Variation) – p. 104
Day 21	Wall Mountain Climbers (Advanced Variation) – p. 34	Wall Squat With Calf Raise – p. 60	Wall-Supported Plank To Pike (Advanced Variation) – p. 72	Wall-Assisted Deep Lunge Stretch (Advanced Variation) – p. 82	Shoulder Blade Squeeze (Advanced Variation) – p. 98
Day 22	Isometric Wall Plank Hold	Glute Bridge Wall Slides	Diamond Wall Push-Ups	Wall-Supported Tree Pose Stretch	Wall Angels – p. 100

	(Advanced Variation) – p. 36	(Advanced Variation) – p. 56	(Advanced Variation) – p. 70	(Advanced Variation) – p. 92	
Day 23	Vertical Wall Sit & Twist – p. 42	Wall Squat Holds (Advanced Variation) – p. 50	Wall Plank Arm Circles – p. 76 (Advanced Variation)	Wall Split Progressions (Advanced Variation) – p. 96	Chin Tucks Against The Wall – p. 102
Day 24	Wall Dead Bug (Advanced Variation) – p. 44	Wall-Supported Pistol Squats (Advanced Variation) – p. 54	Wall Push-Ups (Advanced Variation) – p. 66	Wall-Supported Single Leg Squats (Advanced Variation) – p. 86	Side Wall Arm Stretch (Advanced Variation) – p. 104
Day 25	Wall Leg Raises (Advanced Variation) – p. 38	Elevated Wall Lunges (Advanced Variation) – p. 52	Wall Walks (Advanced Variation) – p. 78	Standing Wall Single-Leg Balance (Advanced Variation) – p. 88	Shoulder Blade Squeeze (Advanced Variation) – p. 98
Day 26	High Wall Knee Tucks (Advanced Variation) – p. 48	Wall Side Leg Lifts (Advanced Variation) – p. 58	Wall Lateral Raise Slides (Advanced Variation) – p. 74	Wall-Supported Warrior III Stretch (Advanced Variation) – p. 90	Wall Angels (Advanced Variation) – p. 100
Day 27	Wall Oblique Crunches (Advanced Variation) – p. 40	Elevated Stallion Pulses (Advanced Variation) – p. 62	Diamond Wall Push-Ups (Advanced Variation) – p. 70	Wall Bridge Extensions (Advanced Variation) – p. 84	Chin Tucks Against The Wall (Advanced Variation) – p. 102
Day 28	Wall Dead Bug With Arm Slide (Advanced Variation) – p. 46	High Wall Glute Kickbacks (Advanced Variation) – p. 64	Wall-Supported Side Plank With Arm Raise (Advanced Variation) – p. 80	Wall Split Progressions (Advanced Variation) – p. 96	Side Wall Arm Stretch (Advanced Variation) – p. 104

CONCLUSION - STAY MOTIVATED

As the final notes of this guide ring in your ears, it's essential to reflect upon the journey you've embarked upon — a journey not just towards physical transformation but holistic well-being. Over the course of this book, we've explored the profound depths of Wall Pilates, an exercise discipline that fuses strength, balance, and grace, choreographing a ballet of movements that promise a revitalized body and spirit.

But this isn't the end. In fact, consider this your beginning.

Every step you've taken, from understanding the basics of Wall Pilates to intricately designing your personalized routines, has been a testament to your commitment. The transformation that you witness in the mirror - the toned glutes, the sculpted abs, the strengthened core, and the upright posture - are the visible symbols of this dedication. Yet, the unseen changes – the surge of self-confidence, the mindfulness in movement, the awakened body awareness – those are the real treasures.

Keeping the Flame Alive

Remaining motivated, especially in the realm of fitness, can be likened to tending a flame. It demands constant care, the right environment, and fuel.

1. Set Evolving Goals: Just as Wall Pilates is about movement, ensure your goals are dynamic too. Once you've achieved a milestone, set the bar a bit higher, always giving yourself something to work towards.

2. Celebrate the Small Wins: Every session completed, every new move mastered, is a victory. Celebrate these moments, not just the broader objectives.

3. Build a Support System: Whether it's joining a Wall Pilates group, finding a workout buddy, or sharing your progress on social platforms – having a supportive community can be the wind beneath your wings.

4. Revisit Your 'Why': On days when the going gets tough, and motivation wanes, remember why you started. Was it to feel healthier? To improve posture? To find a moment of calm in a chaotic day? Reconnect with your 'why'.

Looking Forward

The path of fitness is a marathon, not a sprint. Wall Pilates isn't a trend to be tried and then discarded, but a lifestyle choice, one that requires persistence, dedication, and most importantly, passion. The beauty of Wall Pilates lies in its simplicity and adaptability, making it a discipline that can be woven seamlessly into the fabric of your everyday life.

In this ever-evolving journey, let Wall Pilates be your constant, the anchor amidst life's storms, guiding you towards a harbor of health, happiness, and harmony. As you move forward, remember that every challenge faced is an opportunity for growth, every stumble a lesson learned, and every success, no matter how small, a step closer to the best version of yourself.

To every woman reading this: you possess an innate strength, a reservoir of potential waiting to be tapped. Let Wall Pilates be your guide, your ally in carving out the masterpiece that is you. Welcome the journey, value the process, and allow the magic of Wall Pilates to light your way. Keep advancing, keep growing, and above all, keep having faith. The world is ready for your brilliance. Shine on!

EXCLUSIVE BONUS

First and foremost, Dear Reader, we would like to express our sincere gratitude for starting this life-changing path with "Wall Pilates Workouts for Women." Your dedication to improving physical strength and flexibility, as well as achieving mental clarity and focus, is not just admirable but also a crucial step towards living a more balanced and fulfilling life.

We have some exclusive bonus materials for you as a way of saying thank you and to further enhance your experience. These extras, designed to enhance your journey towards wellness, include:

- **Strategic nutrition to maximizes results**
- **Building your personalized and effective routine**

To claim these valuable resources, just drop us an email at micolipublishing@gmail.com and use the subject line "Wall Pilates Bonus" to ensure your request is handled promptly. Our dedicated team will then send these bonuses directly to your mailbox.

These bonuses are more than just extras; they are a vital component of your path to achieving a balanced body and mind, thoughtfully chosen to complement the skills and knowledge you have gained from the book.

So, don't hesitate! Send us an email right away, and let's unlock these exclusive bonuses!

Printed in Great Britain
by Amazon

37160240R00064